Stress Echocardiography

Stress Echocardiography

Essential Guide and DVD

Edited by

Aleksandar N. Neskovic

Clinical–Hospital Center Zemun
Belgrade University School of Medicine
Belgrade, Serbia

Frank A. Flachskampf

University of Erlangen
Erlangen, Germany

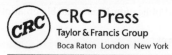

CRC Press
Taylor & Francis Group
Boca Raton London New York

CRC Press is an imprint of the
Taylor & Francis Group, an **informa** business

CRC Press
Taylor & Francis Group
6000 Broken Sound Parkway NW, Suite 300
Boca Raton, FL 33487-2742

First issued in paperback 2019

© 2010 by Taylor & Francis Group, LLC
CRC Press is an imprint of Taylor & Francis Group, an Informa business

No claim to original U.S. Government works

ISBN-13: 978-0-415-42224-6 (hbk)
ISBN-13: 978-0-367-38409-8 (pbk)

A CIP record for this book is available from the British Library.

Library of Congress Cataloging-in-Publication Data available on application

Visit the Taylor & Francis Web site at
http://www.taylorandfrancis.com

and the CRC Press Web site at
http://www.crcpress.com

Preface

Stress echocardiography is a mature clinical tool which in dedicated hands can be immensely useful for patient management. In chronic stable coronary heart disease, research in recent years has shown compellingly that an ischemia-guided management is safe and beneficial for patients. Stress echocardiography is not the only test to identify inducible ischemia, but it is accurate, widely available at relatively low cost, firmly in cardiologists' hands, and radiation-free. It is, however, not an easy technique. Therefore, the editors are delighted to offer the user of this book and DVD a readable, comprehensive, but not encyclopedic introduction to stress echo which is supplemented with a good measure of the most important material to learn stress echo: moving images along with appropriate interpretations. Besides, information on protocols, complications, pitfalls, laboratory organization and many other aspects of the technique are provided by renowned experts in the field who have practiced stress echo for decades. The current applications of stress echo already far exceed the evaluation of chronic coronary artery disease regarding inducible ischemia or contractile reserve and already play an important role in pre-operative risk evaluation, evaluation of the chest pain patient in the emergency room, valvular heart disease, cardiomyopathies, pulmonary hypertension, and other fields.

The editors sincerely hope that the book and DVD will fulfill its purpose to be truly useful introductions to the technique and companions to clinical practice.

Our most sincere gratitude is expressed to the contributors, who offered time, energy, good imaging material, and patience. The editors wish to thank and acknowledge Masha Neskovic, movie director, for her generous and dedicated help in preparation of the video loop files. We also thank very sincerely Joe Stubenrauch and his co-workers from Informa Healthcare who assisted us in the editing process and ensured that everything in the end fell in place.

Aleksandar N. Neskovic
Frank A. Flachskampf

Contents

Contributors

Maria Joao Andrade Hospital de Santa Cruz, Lisbon, Portugal

Georges Athanassopoulos Onassis Cardiac Surgery Center, Athens, Greece

Manish Bansal University of Queensland, Brisbane, Australia

Navtej S. Chahal Department of Cardiology, Northwick Park Hospital, Harrow, U.K.

Paolo Colonna Institute of Cardiology, Policlinico Hospital, Bari, Italy

Vojkan Cvorovic Department of Cardiology, Clinical-Hospital Center Zemun, Belgrade University School of Medicine, Belgrade, Serbia

Anai E. Durazzo Department of Vascular Surgery, Erasmus Medical Centre, Rotterdam, The Netherlands

Frank A. Flachskampf Medizinische Klinik 2, University of Erlangen, Erlangen, Germany

Andreas Hagendorff Department of Cardiology-Angiology, University of Leipzig, Leipzig, Germany

Sanne E. Hoeks Department of Anaesthesiology, Erasmus Medical Centre, Rotterdam, The Netherlands

Thomas H. Marwick University of Queensland, Brisbane, Australia

Aleksandar N. Neskovic Department of Cardiology, Clinical-Hospital Center Zemun, Belgrade University School of Medicine, Belgrade, Serbia

Eugenio Picano CNR, Institute of Clinical Physiology, Pisa, Italy

Don Poldermans Department of Vascular Surgery, Erasmus Medical Centre, Rotterdam, The Netherlands

Bogdan A. Popescu "Carol Davila" University of Medicine and Pharmacy, and "C. C. Iliescu" Institute of Cardiovascular Diseases, Bucharest, Romania

Biljana Putnikovic Department of Cardiology, Clinical-Hospital Center Zemun, Belgrade University School of Medicine, Belgrade, Serbia

Leonardo Rodriguez Cardiovascular Imaging Center, Heart and Vascular Institute, Cleveland Clinic, Cleveland, Ohio, U.S.A.

Roxy Senior   Department of Cardiology, Northwick Park Hospital, Harrow, U.K.

Rosa Sicari   CNR, Institute of Clinical Physiology, Pisa, Italy

Alja Vlahovic-Stipac   Department of Cardiology, Clinical-Hospital Center Zemun, Belgrade University School of Medicine, Belgrade, Serbia

1 Basic Principles of Stress Echocardiography: Why, When and How?

Eugenio Picano

CNR, Institute of Clinical Physiology, Pisa, Italy

Stress echocardiography is the combination of two-dimensional echocardiography with a physical, pharmacological, or electrical stress (1). The diagnostic endpoint for detection of myocardial ischemia is the induction of a transient change in regional left ventricular function during stress. The stress echo sign of ischemia is a stress-induced worsening of function in a region contracting normally at baseline. The stress echo sign of myocardial viability is instead a stress-induced improvement of function in a region that is abnormal at rest (Fig. 1; Table 1). Stress-induced ST-segment depression is not per se a criterion of test positivity, since it can be frequently found in the absence of wall motion abnormalities with angiographically normal coronary arteries, in the so-called microvascular coronary artery disease frequently found in women, hypertensives, and diabetics (2) (Fig. 2).

I. WHY STRESS ECHO? A HISTORICAL, PATHOPHYSIOLOGICAL AND SOCIETAL PERSPECTIVE

In 1935, Tennant and Wiggers demonstrated that coronary occlusion immediately resulted in instantaneous abnormality of wall motion (3). Experimental studies performed some 40 years later on the canine model with ultrasonic crystals and two-dimensional echocardiography proved that during acute ischemia (4) and infarction (5), reductions in regional flow are closely mirrored by reductions in contractile functions, and set the stage for clinical use of ultrasonic methods in ischemic heart disease. The regional wall motion abnormality is an early event in the ischemic cascade—and also a very specific signal of myocardial ischemia (Fig. 2).

The very first reports describing echocardiographic changes during ischemia dealt with the use of M-mode techniques in exercise-induced (6) and vasospastic, variant angina (7). These studies recognized, for the first time, transient dyssynergy to be an early, sensitive, specific marker of transient ischemia, clearly more accurate than echocardiography changes and pain. The clinical impact of the technique became more obvious in the mid-1980s with the combination of two-dimensional echocardiography with pharmacological stress, represented by dipyridamole (8) or dobutamine (9)—both much less technically demanding than post–treadmill exercise commonly used in the United States (10).

Stress echocardiography has evolved in Europe in a significantly different fashion from that in the United States. Pharmacological stress echo has been

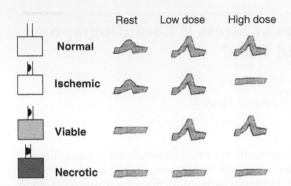

FIGURE 1   Echocardiographic examples of two-dimensional–targeted M-mode tracings of normal (*upper row*), ischemic (*second row*), viable (*third row*), and necrotic (*fourth row*) responses. In a normal segment, the segment increases both at low and high doses with a normal hyperkinetic response (*top row*). In an ischemic segment perfused by a significant coronary stenosis, the function is normal at rest but worsens at peak stress (*second row*). In a viable myocardium with resting dysfunction and fed by a coronary artery with noncritical coronary stenosis, the segment is hypokinetic or akinetic at rest and normokinetic during stress (*third row*). Necrotic tissue shows unchanged function throughout the test, regardless of the underlying anatomical condition of the infarct-related vessel (*fourth row*).

widely accepted in clinical practice, and this has allowed to collect a tremendous amount of data from large-scale, multicenter, effective studies, allowing to establish the safety and prognostic value of stress echo on thousands of patients studied under the "real world conditions" (11,12). In European clinical practice, stress echo had to be embedded under the legal and cultural framework of the existing European laws and medical imaging referral guidelines. Use of radiation for medical examinations and tests is the largest man-made source of radiation exposure (13). Small individual risks of each test performed with ionizing radiation multiplied by billion examinations become significant population risks. For this reason, in Europe, both the law (14) and the referral guidelines for medical imaging (15) recommend a justified, optimized, and responsible use of testing with ionizing radiation. The Euratom Directive 97/43 establishes that the indication and execution of diagnostic procedures with ionizing radiation should follow three basic principles: the justification principle (article 3: "if an exposure cannot be justified, it should be prohibited"), the optimization principle (article 4: according to ALARA principle, "all doses due to medical exposures must be kept As Low As Reasonably Achievable"), and the responsibility principle (article 5: "both the prescriber and the practitioner are responsible for the justification of the test exposing the patient to ionising

TABLE 1   Stress Echocardiography in Four Equations

Rest	+	Stress	=	Diagnosis
Normokinesis	+	Normokinesis, Hyperkinesis	=	Normal
Normokinesis	+	Hypokinesis, Akinesis, Dyskinesis	=	Ischemia
Akinesis	+	Hypokinesis, Normokinesis	=	Viable
Akinesis, Dyskinesis	+	Akinesis, Dyskinesis	=	Necrosis

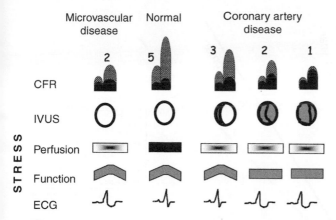

FIGURE 2 A synthetic view of the different pathophysiological situations of classic (coronary artery disease) and alternative (microvascular) ischemic cascade. In the normal condition (*framed, second column from left*), there is a normal coronary flow reserve (CFR; *first row*, with intracoronary Doppler ultrasound), normal coronary anatomy, normal perfusion pattern with scintigraphy (perfusion, *second row*), and normal contraction during stress (function, *third row*). Coronary flow reserve is pictorially expressed with a transthoracic pulsed Doppler tracing sampled on mid-distal left anterior descending coronary artery. With classical ischemic cascade, perfusion defects are present with mild (*third column from the right*), moderate (*second column from the right*), and severe (*first column from the right*) coronary stenosis, mirroring reductions in coronary flow reserve and accompanied (for moderate-to-severe stenoses) by regional wall motion abnormalities, which are usually absent for mild degrees of stenosis, capable to limit coronary flow reserve without inducing ischemia. In microvascular disease (*first column from the left*), the depressed coronary flow reserve is associated with a normal coronary anatomy, the frequent occurrence of stress-induced perfusion defects (often with ST-segment depression), and normal left ventricular function. *Abbreviations*: CFR, coronary flow reserve; IVUS, intravascular ultrasound. *Source*: From Ref. 2.

radiation"). European Commission referral guidelines were released in 2001 in application of Euratom Directive and explicitly state that a nonionizing technique must be used whenever it will give grossly comparable information to an ionizing investigation. For instance, "because MRI does not use ionizing radiation, MRI should be preferred when both CT and MRI would provide similar information and when both are available" (14).

In the field of cardiac stress imaging, this translates very clearly in a privileged choice of stress echo instead of stress perfusion scintigraphy, which gives a radiation exposure per test ranging from 500 chest X-rays (sestamibi) to 1600 chest X-rays (thallium or dual isotope scintigraphy) (Fig. 3). This gives an extra risk per patient of 1 cancer every 400 (for thallium) to 1000 (for sestamibi) exposed patients. The situation is not better if we move from an individual to a society perspective (16). About 10 million perfusion stress testing are performed each year in the United States, corresponding to a population risk of 20,000 lifetime new cancers each year. There is a little doubt that a diagnostic flowchart centered on stress echo as a first choice and stress MRI in selected cases would dramatically benefit the social long-term damages associated with cardiac stress testing (17). In this perspective of the medical, as well as societal and biological impact of medical imaging, it is imperative to increase all efforts

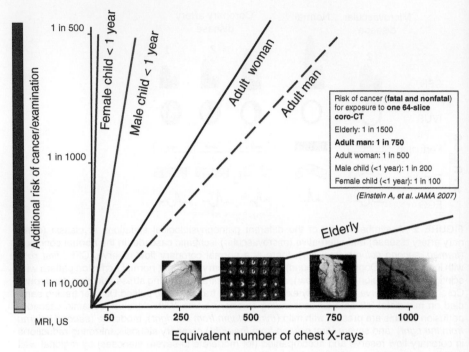

FIGURE 3   (*See color insert*) Doses and risks of cardiac stress testing. The dose equivalent of a cardiac stress scintigraphy ranges from 500 chest X-rays (sestamibi) to 1250 chest X-rays (thallium) to 1700 chest X-rays (dual isotope). The corresponding risk of cancer for a 50-year-old man ranges from 1 in 1000 (sestamibi) to 1 in 400 (dual isotope). Doses of other common procedures, such as coronary angiography (250 chest X-rays), multislice cardiac CT (750 chest X-rays), and coronary stenting (1000 chest X-rays) are shown for comparison. *Source*: From Ref. 19.

to improve appropriateness (18) and to minimize the radiation burden of stress imaging for the population and the individual patient (17). The imperative of sustainability of medical imaging is likely to become increasingly important in the near future, also from a U.S. perspective (15,16). In the quest of sustainability, stress echocardiography has unsurpassed assets of low cost, absence of environmental impact, lack of biological effects for both the patient (19), and the operator when evaluated against equally accurate, but less sustainable, competing techniques (20).

II.   WHEN STRESS ECHO? INDICATIONS

Imaging test (including stress echo) cannot be used as a first-line technique, but should be limited to patients with ambiguous or nondiagnostic or inconclusive results on exercise-echocardiography stress test (Fig. 4). In fact, even though exercise electrocardiography is less sensitive and feasible than stress echocardiography, the negative predictive value of maximal test is high and a negative maximal exercise electrocardiography test identifies a large group of patients at low risk with annual hard events rate <1%. It is very difficult for any imaging stress to add further information to this subset. On the other end of the spectrum, a

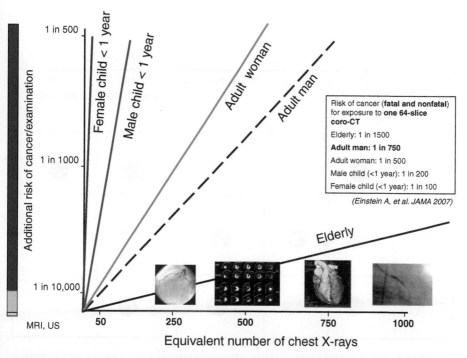

FIGURE 1.3 Doses and risks of cardiac stress testing. The dose equivalent of a cardiac stress scintigraphy ranges from 500 chest X-rays (sestamibi) to 1250 chest X-rays (thallium) to 1700 chest X-rays (dual isotope). The corresponding risk of cancer for a 50-year-old man ranges from 1 in 1000 (sestamibi) to 1 in 400 (dual isotope). Doses of other common procedures, such as coronary angiography (250 chest X-rays), multislice cardiac CT (750 chest X-rays), and coronary stenting (1000 chest X-rays) are shown for comparison. *Source*: From Ref. 19.

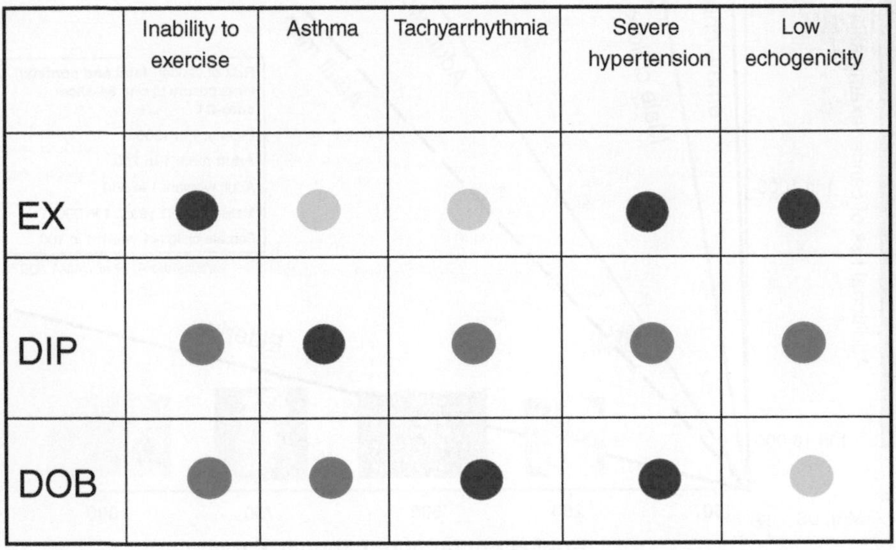

	Inability to exercise	Asthma	Tachyarrhythmia	Severe hypertension	Low echogenicity
EX	●	○	○	●	●
DIP	●	●	●	●	●
DOB	●	●	●	●	○

FIGURE 1.5 The right type of stress echocardiography (exercise, dipyridamole, or dobutamine) can be chosen according to several clinical and resting echocardiography variables.

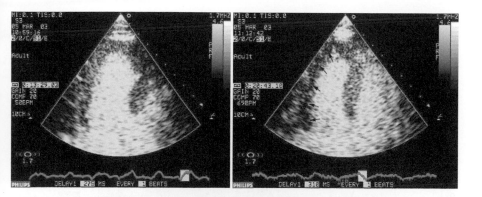

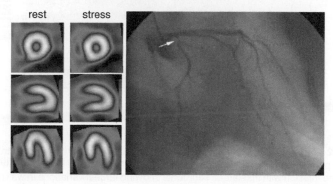

FIGURE 8.7 MCE on a patient at rest (*left*; loop 65) and with stress (*right*; loop 66). There is a clear subendocardial perfusion defect in the circumflex artery territory (*black arrows*). Radionuclide uptake on SPECT was normal. Coronary angiography confirmed the presence of a flow-limiting lesion in the circumflex artery (loop 67).

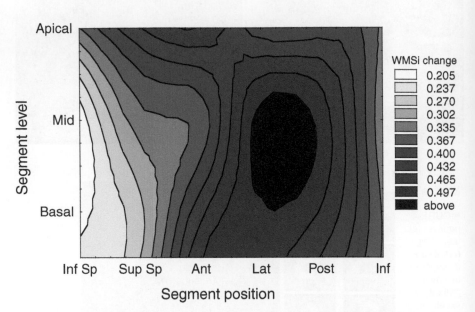

FIGURE 10.2 Segmental variations of wall motion score index during dobutamin stress echocardiography in patients with idiopathic dilated cardiomyopathy. Regional heterogeneity in response to dobutamine infusion with mid-lateral segments showing largest variations in wall motion score index can be noted. *Abbreviation*: WMSi, wall motion score index. *Source*: From Ref. 23.

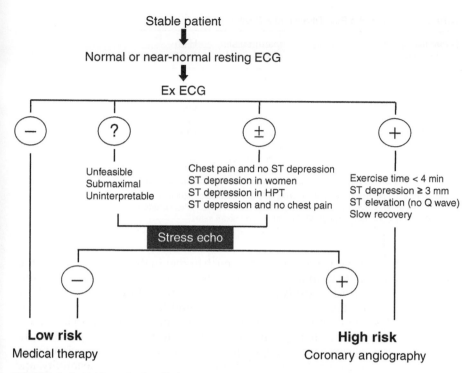

FIGURE 4 In stable patients with known or suspected coronary artery disease and normal or near-normal resting ECG, the diagnostic algorithm should start with exercise electrocardiography test. This remains the first noninvasive test to be done and often the last one: a maximal negative test is associated with an extremely good prognosis; on the other end of the spectrum, a response of severe ischemia warrants coronary angiography without further investigations. In patients with ambiguous or uninterpretable results during exercise electrocardiography or patients in whom exercise is submaximal or contraindicated, stress echocardiography is an excellent choice. A negative stress echo identifies a low-risk group. A positive stress echo warrants a more aggressive therapeutic approach. *Source*: From Ref. 22.

high-risk response (with low workload positivity, exercise-induced hypertension, slow recovery) identifies a group at high risk in which an imaging test might be redundant; this subset of patients has to be treated in an aggressive way. Stress echocardiography yields the greatest incremental diagnostic and prognostic value in patients who had a nondiagnostic, or ambiguous, or inconclusive exercise electrocardiography (21–30). Pharmacological stress echocardiography is the obligatory choice in patients in whom exercise is unfeasible or contraindicated. The choice of one pharmacological test over the other as the preferred imaging modality may depend upon local drug cost, tests safety, and expertise available. Vasodilator, inotropic, and exercise stresses are all needed to optimize the enormous diagnostic and prognostic potential of echocardiography in a modern stress echo laboratory. In patients with permanent pacemaker, noninvasive pacemaker stress echo is an excellent choice (31). Whatever be the test choice, the results of physical or pharmacological stress echo should be used as a "gatekeeper" to coronary angiography. In fact, for any given coronary anatomy, the

TABLE 2 Stress Echo Risk Titration of a Positive Test

1-Year risk (hard events)	Intermediate (1–3% year)	High (>10% year)
Dose/workload	High	Low
Resting EF	>50%	<40%
Anti-ischemic therapy	Off	On
Coronary territory	LCx/RCA	LAD
Peak WMSI	Low	High
Recovery	Fast	Slow
Positivity or baseline dyssynergy	Homozonal	Heterozonal
CFR	>2.0	<2.0

Abbreviations: CFR, coronary flow reserve; EF, left ventricular ejection fraction; LAD, left anterior descending coronary artery; LCx, left circumflex coronary artery; RCA, right coronary artery; WMSI, wall motion score index.

prognostic benefit of revascularization is much higher in the presence of ischemia documented on stress testing. Patients with stress echo positivity, and especially those with a "high-risk" positivity pattern (occurring at low dose of workload, under anti-ischemic therapy, with slow recovery and/or antidote resistance, with akinesia or dyskinesia of more than five segments of the left ventricle) should be referred to coronary angiography (Table 2). By applying this algorithm, the number of useless coronary angiographies and costly revascularization procedures would be substantially reduced. Patients with stress echo negativity, and especially those with a "very low risk" negativity pattern (i.e., off anti-ischemic therapy, with normal resting left ventricular function and maximal stress) should be kept on medical therapy.

When technology and expertise allow, stress echo will increase its diagnostic and—most critically—prognostic potential through the simultaneous evaluation of wall motion and coronary flow reserve of mid-distal left anterior descending coronary artery by pulsed Doppler during vasodilator stress (32). Patients with negative wall motion criteria, with relatively high-risk clinical features, such as concomitant anti-ischemic therapy at the time of testing (32), diabetes (33), or dilated cardiomyopathy (34), can be further separated on the basis of coronary flow reserve. Anti-ischemic therapy at the time of testing prevents ischemia and development of wall motion abnormalities through an antisteal effect, improving subendocardial perfusion at any given transmural flow (35), but affects much less the coronary flow reserve (36,37). If a patient with negative wall motion has also a preserved coronary flow reserve above 2.0, the outcome is excellent also on the long run, since there is integrity of the epicardial vessels determining not only wall motion abnormalities but also the coronary microcirculation mirrored in coronary flow reserve (Table 3).

III. HOW TO DO STRESS ECHO? CONTRAINDICATIONS

The absolute and relative contraindications to stress testing are summarized in Table 4, together with selective indications to specific forms of stress. Obviously, a poor acoustic window makes any form of stress echocardiography unfeasible. However, a difficult resting echocardiography greatly increases the probability of

TABLE 3 Stress Echo Risk Titration of a Negative Test

1-Year risk (hard events)	Very low (<0.5% year)	Low (1–3% year)
Stress	Maximal	Submaximal
Resting EF	>50%	<40%
Anti-ischemic therapy	Off	On
CFR	>2.0	<2.0

Abbreviations: CFR, coronary flow reserve; EF, left ventricular ejection fraction.

obtaining no interpretable study results during exercise and should be an indication for the less technically demanding pharmacological stress echocardiography to be used (Fig. 5). Specific contraindications to dipyridamole (or adenosine) echocardiography include the presence of severe conduction disturbances, as adenosine can cause transient conduction block, and severe bronchospasm requiring chronic xanthine therapy, as adenosine is a powerful bronchoconstrictor. Patients with resting systolic blood pressure under 100 mm Hg generally should not receive dobutamine or dipyridamole. Dobutamine not only causes an increase in systolic blood pressure in the majority of patients but can also cause a significant decrease in systolic blood pressure in a substantial minority of patients. Dipyridamole usually causes a modest decrease in systolic blood pressure of 10 to 20 mm Hg, but occasionally causes a more severe decrease. Adenosine is the preferred option because of its rapid half-life (<10 sec) in patients with unstable carotid artery disease. Significant hypertension and prolonged hypotension should be avoided in these patients, making adenosine the agent of choice. Patients who do not achieve the target heart rate with dobutamine alone or inducible ischemia with dipyridamole alone are commonly administered atropine. Atropine use in this setting is a risk only for closed-angle

TABLE 4 Stress Echo: Which Test for Which Patient?

Patient characteristics	Exercise	Dipyridamole	Dobutamine
Inability to exercise	3	1	1
Contraindication to exercise	3	1	1
Positive EET at ≤6 min of exercise in hypertensives, women, baseline ECG changes	1	2	2
Asthmatic patient	2	3	1
Under theophylline therapy	1	3	1
Severe hypertension	3	1	3
Well-controlled hypertension	2	1	2
Relative hypotension	1	3	3
Ventricular ectopy	1	1	3
2nd-3rd degree AV block	1	3	2
Suboptimal acoustic window	3	1	2
Evaluation of anti-ischemic therapy efficacy	1	2	3
Unstable carotid disease	2	2	2
Permanent pacemaker	Pacemaker stress ECHO		

1, especially indicated; 2, relatively contraindicated; 3, contraindicated.
Abbreviation: EET, exercise ECG test.

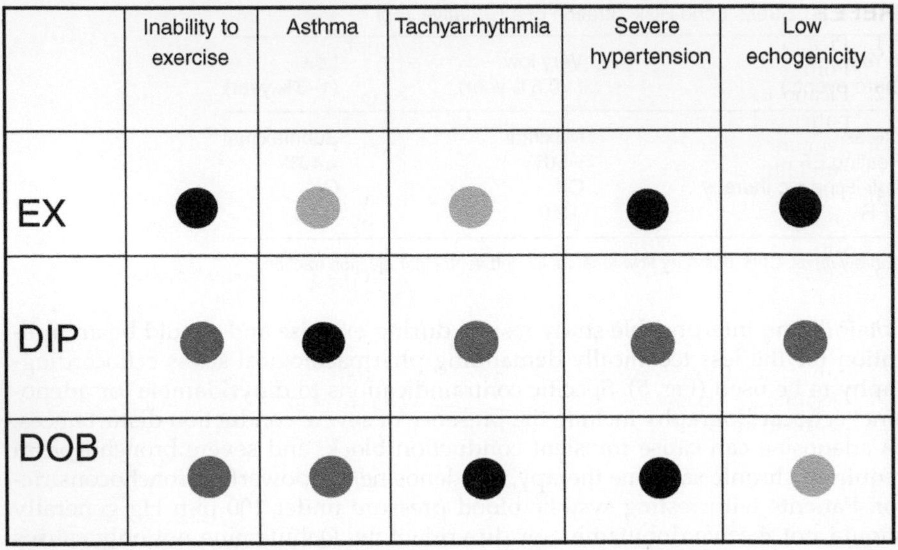

	Inability to exercise	Asthma	Tachyarrhythmia	Severe hypertension	Low echogenicity
EX	●	●	●	●	●
DIP	●	●	●	●	●
DOB	●	●	●	●	●

FIGURE 5 (*See color insert*) The right type of stress echocardiography (exercise, dipyridamole, or dobutamine) can be chosen according to several clinical and resting echocardiography variables.

glaucoma patients, a minority of patients with glaucoma. If eye pain occurs, the patient should call an ophthalmologist the same day. Severe prostate disease is also a contraindication to atropine use.

IV. CONCLUSION

Recent European Society of Cardiology guidelines clearly state that stress echocardiography provides similar diagnostic and prognostic accuracy as radionuclide stress perfusion imaging (38), but at a substantially lower cost, without environmental impact, and with no biohazards for the patient and the physician. Different stresses (exercise, dipyridamole, dobutamine) have comparable diagnostic and prognostic accuracy—according to evidence-based medicine mirrored in European guidelines. Semisupine exercise is the most used, dobutamine is the best test for viability, and dipyridamole is the safest and the simplest pharmacological stress and the most suitable for combined wall motion—coronary flow reserve assessment (39,40). The additional clinical benefit of new technologies such as tissue Doppler and strain rate imaging has been inconsistent and disappointing (39,40), whereas the potential of adding coronary flow reserve evaluation of left anterior descending coronary artery by transthoracic Doppler echocardiography adds another potentially important dimension to stress echocardiography (39). Despite its dependence upon operator's training (41), stress echocardiography is today the best possible imaging choice to achieve the still elusive target of sustainable cardiac imaging in the field of noninvasive diagnosis of coronary artery disease.

DVD note: The following loops are related to the content of this chapter: 1–33. These loops can be found in the provided DVD.

REFERENCES

1. Picano E. Stress echocardiography: From pathophysiological toy to diagnostic tool. Point of view. Circulation 1992; 85:1604–1612.
2. Picano E, Palinkas A, Amyot R. Diagnosis of myocardial ischemia in hypertensive patients. J Hypert 2001; 19:1177–1183.
3. Tennant R, Wiggers CJ. The effects of coronary occlusion on myocardial contraction. Am J Physiol 1935; 112:351–361.
4. Theroux P, Franklin D, Ross J Jr, et al. Regional myocardial function during acute coronary artery occlusion and its modification by pharmacologic agents in the dog. Circ Res 1974; 34:896–908.
5. Kerber RE, Abboud FM. Echocardiographic detection of regional myocardial infarction. An experimental study. Circulation 1973; 47:997–1005.
6. Sugishita Y, Koseki S, Matsuda M, et al. Dissociation between regional myocardial dysfunction and ECG changes during myocardial ischemia induced by exercise in patients with angina pectoris. Am Heart J 1983; 106:1–8.
7. Distante A, Rovai D, Picano E, et al. Transient changes in left ventricular mechanics during attacks of Prinzmetal's angina: An M-mode echocardiographic study. Am Heart J 1984; 107:465–470.
8. Picano E, Distante A, Masini M, et al. Dipyridamole-echocardiography test in effort angina pectoris. Am J Cardiol 1985; 56:452–456.
9. Pierard LA, De Landshcere CM, Berthe C, et al. Identification of viable myocardium by echocardiography during dobutamine infusion in patients with myocardial infarction after thrombolytic therapy: Comparison with positron emission tomography. J Am Coll Cardiol 1990; 15:1021–1031.
10. Wann LS, Faris JV, Childress RH, et al. Exercise cross-sectional echocardiography in ischemic heart disease. Circulation 1979; 60:1300–1308.
11. Picano E, Mathias W Jr, Pingitore A, et al. Safety and tolerability of dobutamine-atropine stress echocardiography: A prospective, multicentre study Echo Dobutamine International Cooperative Study Group. Lancet 1994; 344:1190–1192.
12. Picano E, Sicari R, Landi P, et al.; for the EDIC Study Group Prognostic value of myocardial viability in medically treated patients with global left ventricular dysfunction early after an acute uncomplicated myocardial infarction: A dobutamine stress echocardiographic study. Circulation 1998; 98:1078–1084.
13. Council Directive 97/43/Euratom of 30 June 1997 on health protection of individuals against the dangers of ionising radiation in relation to medical exposure, and repealing Directive 84/466/Euratom. Official Journal No. L 180, 09/07/1997 P. 0022–0027.
14. European Commission Referral Guidelines for imaging. Rad Protect 2001; 118:1–125. Available at: http://europa.eu.int/comm/environment/radprot/118/rp-118-en.pdf (accessed July 28, 2007).
15. Picano E. Sustainability of medical imaging. Education and Debate. BMJ 2004; 328:578–580.
16. Amis ES Jr, Butler PF, Applegate KE, et al. American College of Radiology white paper on radiation dose in medicine. J Am Coll Radiol 2007; 4:272–284.
17. Picano E, Vano E, Semelka R, et al. The American College of Radiology white paper on radiation dose in medicine: Deep impact on the practice of cardiovascular imaging. Cardiovasc Ultrasound 2007; 5:37.
18. Picano E, Pasanisi E, Brown J, et al. A gatekeeper for the gatekeeper; inappropriate referrals to stress echocardiography. Am Heart J 2007; 154:126–132.
19. Picano E. Informed consent in radiological and nuclear medicine examinations. How to escape from a communication Inferno. Education and debate. BMJ 2004; 329:578–580.
20. Picano E. Stress echocardiography: A historical perspective. Special article. Am J Med 2003; 114:126–130.
21. Picano E, Severi S, Michelassi C, et al. Prognostic importance of dipyridamole-echocardiography test in coronary artery disease. Circulation 1989; 80:450–459.

22. Severi S, Picano E, Michelassi C, et al. Diagnostic and prognostic value of dipyridamole echocardiography in patients with suspected coronary artery disease: Comparison with exercise electrocardiography. Circulation 1994; 89:1160–1173.
23. Sicari R, Ripoli A, Picano E, et al.; on behalf of the EPIC Study Group. Perioperative prognostic value of dipyridamole echocardiography in vascular surgery: A large scale multicenter study on 509 patients. Circulation 1999; 100:II269–II274.
24. Sicari R, Cortigiani L, Bigi R, et al.; on behalf of the Echo-Persantine International Cooperative (EPIC) and Echo-Dobutamine International Cooperative (EDIC) Study Groups. The prognostic value of pharmacological stress echo is affected by concomitant anti-ischemic therapy at the time of testing. Circulation 2004; 109:2428.
25. Cortigiani L, Paolini EA, Nannini E. Dipyridamole stress echocardiography for risk stratification in hypertensive patients with chest pain. Circulation 1998; 98:2855–2859.
26. Cortigiani L, Picano E, Landi P, et al. Value of pharmacological stress echocardiography in risk stratification of patients with single-vessel disease. A report from the echo-persantine and echo-dobutamine international cooperative studies. J Am Coll Cardiol 1998; 32:69–74.
27. Cortigiani L, Bigi R, Sicari R, et al. Prognostic value of pharmacological stress echocardiography in diabetic and nondiabetic patients with known or suspected coronary artery disease. J Am Coll Cardiol 2006; 47:605–610.
28. Marwick TH, Case C, Vasey C, et al. Prediction of mortality by exercise echocardiography: A strategy for combination with the duke treadmill score. Circulation 2001; 103:2566–2571.
29. Marwick TH, Case C, Sawada S, et al. Prediction of mortality using dobutamine echocardiography. J Am Coll Cardiol 2001; 37:754–760.
30. Poldermans D, Fioretti PM, Forster T, et al. Dobutamine stress echocardiography for assessment of perioperative cardiac risk in patients undergoing major vascular surgery. Circulation 1993; 87:1506–1512.
31. Picano E, Alaimo A, Chubuchny V, et al. Noninvasive pacemaker stress echocardiography for diagnosis of coronary artery disease: A multicenter study. J Am Coll Cardiol 2002; 40:1305–1310.
32. Rigo F, Cortigiani L, Pasanisi E, et al. The additional prognostic value of coronary flow reserve on left anterior descending artery in patients with negative stress echo by wall motion criteria. A transthoracic vasodilator stress echocardiography study. Am Heart J 2006; 151:124–130.
33. Cortigiani L, Rigo F, Gherardi S, et al. Additional prognostic value of coronary flow reserve in diabetic and nondiabetic patients with negative dipyridamole stress echocardiography by wall motion criteria. J Am Coll Cardiol 2007; 50:1354–1361.
34. Rigo F, Gherardi S, Galderisi M, et al. The prognostic impact of coronary flow-reserve assessed by Doppler echocardiography in non-ischaemic dilated cardiomyopathy. Eur Heart J 2006; 27:1319–1323.
35. Lattanzi F, Picano E, Bolognese L, et al. Inhibition of dipyridamole-induced ischemia by antianginal therapy in humans. Correlation with exercise echocardiography. Circulation 1991; 83:1256–1262.
36. Rigo F, Sicari R, Gherardi S, et al. The additive prognostic value of wall motion abnormalities and coronary flow reserve during dipyridamole stress echo therapy. Eur Heart J 2008; 29:79–88.
37. Sicari R, Rigo F, Gherardi S, et al. The prognostic value of Doppler echocardiographic-derived coronary flow reserve is not affected by concomitant antiischemic therapy at the time of testing. Am Heart J 2008; 156:573–579.
38. Fox K, Garcia MA, Ardissino D, et al. Task Force on the Management of Stable Angina Pectoris of the European Society of Cardiology; ESC Committee for Practice Guidelines (CPG), Guidelines on the management of stable angina pectoris: Executive summary: The Task Force on the Management of Stable Angina Pectoris of the European Society of Cardiology.

39. Sicari R, Nihoyannopoulos P, Evangelista A, et al. Stress echocardiography expert consensus statement from the European association of echocardiography. Eur J Echocardiogr 2008; 9:415–437.
40. Pellikka PA, Nague SF, Elhendy AA, et al. American Society of Echocardiography recommendations for performance, interpretation, and application of stress echocardiography. J Am Soc Echocardiogr 2007; 20:1021–1041.
41. Picano E. Lattanzi F, Orlandini A, et al. Stress echocardiography and the human factor: The importance of being expert. J Am Coll Cardiol 1991; 17:666–669.

Stress and Stressors: Applied Pathophysiology

Eugenio Picano
CNR, Institute of Clinical Physiology, Pisa, Italy

Stresses have different pathophysiological and clinical targets (Table 1): coronary vasospasm; coronary artery stenosis; coronary flow reserve in high-risk patients with normal coronary arteries and negative wall motion response during stress echocardiography; identification of viable myocardium with resting dysfunction; assessment of severity of valvular heart disease in special subsets, such as low-gradient aortic stenosis and mitral stenosis with discordant symptoms and stenosis severity; identification of vulnerability to development of pulmonary hypertension. Each clinical target has a distinct echocardiographic diagnostic marker and a preferred stress. Tests inducing vasospasm (ergometrine infusion and hyperventilation) explore the functional component of myocardial ischemia. Tests targeting coronary stenosis (exercise, dipyridamole or adenosine, dobutamine, pacing) mostly explore the ceiling of coronary reserve as defined by organic factors. Viability stresses elicit a contractile response in myocardium with resting dysfunction through an inotropic challenge, primarily focused on myocyte (dobutamine or enoximone or low-level exercise) or mediated by an increase in coronary flow (dipyridamole or nitroglycerine). Coronary flow reserve is best studied with selective and powerful coronary vasodilators capable of fully recruiting microcirculatory vasodilatory capacity. Valvular function in aortic or mitral stenoses can be challenged with stresses increasing cardiac output and therefore transvalvular flow, which determines a steep increase in transvalvular gradients in functionally more severe stenosis. Finally, a vasoconstriction of pulmonary vasculature can be elicited only with exercise, leading to the identification of subjects with normal resting values of pulmonary artery systolic pressure, but vulnerable to developing genetically or environmentally mediated pulmonary hypertension.

I. ISCHEMIA AND VASOSPASM

The smooth muscle cell in the medial layer of coronary epicardial arteries reacts to several vasoconstrictive stimuli, coming centripetally from the adventitial layer (such as alpha-mediated vasoconstriction), or centrifugally from the intima–blood interface (such as endothelin and serotonin). In fact, serotonin has a vasodilator effect on normal human myocardial arteries, which is mediated by endothelium-derived relaxing factors; when the endothelium is damaged, as in coronary artery disease, serotonin has a direct, unopposed vasoconstrictive effect (2). Clinically, coronary vasospasm can be elicited by ergometrine, an ergot alkaloid that stimulates both α-adrenergic and serotonergic receptors, and therefore exerts a direct constrictive effect on vascular smooth muscle (Fig. 1).

TABLE 1 Clinical Targets: Coronary Artery Disease, Dilated Cardiomyopathy, Valvular Disease, and Pulmonary Hypertension

Clinical condition	Pathophysiological target	Stress of choice	Echo variable
Variant angina	Coronary vasospasm	Ergo, Hyperv	WM
Coronary artery disease	Myocardial ischemia	Ex, Dob, Dip	WM
Dilated cardiomyopathy	Contractile reserve	Dob (Ex, Dip)	WM
Diabetes, hypertension, HCM	Coronary flow reserve	Dip (Dob, Ex)	PW LAD
Transmitral gradient	Increase in cardiac output	Ex, Dob	PW mitral
Transaortic gradient	Increase in cardiac output	Ex, Dob	CW aortic
Pulmonary hypertension	Pulmonary vasoconstriction	Ex	CW TR

Abbreviations: CW, continuous wave Doppler; Dob, dobutamine; Dip, dipyridamole; Ex, exercise; HCM, hypertrophic cardiomyopathy; Hyperv, hyperventilation; LAD, left anterior descending coronary artery; PW, pulsed wave Doppler; TR, tricuspid regurgitation; WM, wall motion.

Hyperventilation induces spasm through systemic alkalosis. Physiologically, a powerful calcium-antagonistic action is exerted by hydrogen ions, which seem to compete with calcium ions for the same active sites both in the transmembrane calcium transport system and in the myofibrillar ATPase. Thus, vasoconstriction occurs if either calcium ion concentration increases or hydrogen ion concentration decreases. Exercise can also induce an increase of coronary tone, up to complete vasospasm, through alpha-sympathetic stimulation. Dobutamine has a vasospastic and coronary vasoconstrictive effect mediated by α-adrenergic stimulation (3). Dipyridamole per se has no coronary constrictive effects; however, interruption of the test by aminophylline (which not only blocks adenosine receptors but also stimulates α-adrenoreceptors) can evoke coronary vasospasm in one-third of the patients with variant angina (4). It is important to recognize vasospasm not only through targeted testing but also when it appears by serendipity, that is, as an unexpected manifestation of testing focused on coronary artery stenosis (typically, a sudden positivity with ST-segment elevation in

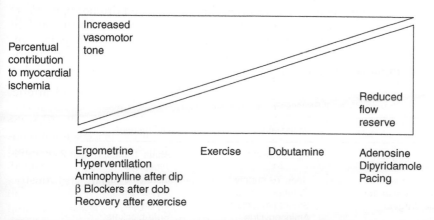

FIGURE 1 Conceptual allocation of the tests employed in combination with echocardiography to induce ischemia via coronary vasospasm (*left*), coronary stenosis (*right*), or both mechanisms. *Source*: From Ref. 1.

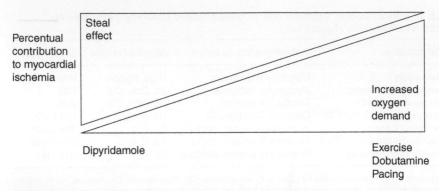

FIGURE 2 Conceptual allocation of tests employed in combination with echocardiography to detect coronary artery stenosis inducing ischemia via steal effect (*left*) or increased myocardial oxygen demand (*right*), or both mechanisms. *Source*: From Ref. 1.

the recovery phase of an otherwise negative exercise, dobutamine, and dipyridamole stress) (Fig. 1).

II. ISCHEMIA AND ORGANIC CORONARY DISEASE

Tests exploring organic coronary stenosis can induce ischemia by two basic mechanisms: (a) an increase in oxygen demand, exceeding the fixed supply; (b) flow maldistribution due to inappropriate coronary arteriolar vasodilation triggered by a metabolic/pharmacological stimulus (Fig. 2). The main pharmacodynamic actions of dobutamine and dipyridamole stresses are summarized in Table 2. Dobutamine has complex dose-dependent effects on β_1- and β_2- and α_1-adrenoreceptors (5), whereas the principal target of adenosine and dipyridamole are adenosine receptors, both A_1 and A_2, present both in myocardium and coronary vessels (6). In particular, stimulation of A_2a receptors produces marked dilation of coronary resistance vessels, determining arteriolar vasodilation, whereas A_2b receptors mediate vasodilation in conductance vessels. Myocardial A_1 adenosine receptors mediate the negative chronotropic and dromotropic effects of adenosine and the direct algogenic effect. A_3 receptors are found on the surface of mast cells and may play a role in mediating bronchospasm and hypotension. Exogenous and endogenous adenosine may profoundly dilate coronary arterioles with minimal effect, if any, on systemic circulation, probably because A_2a

TABLE 2 Pharmacological Stresses

	Vasodilator	Dobutamine
Receptor targets	A₂ adenosine	Alpha 1; beta 1; beta 2 adrenoreceptors
Hemodynamic mechanisms	Reduces supply	Increases supply
Physiological targets	Coronary arterioles	Myocardium
Cellular targets	Smooth muscle cells	Myocytes
Antidote	Aminophylline	Beta-blockers
Stress	Dipyridamole (adenosine)	Dobutamine
Contraindications	Asthma, bradyarrhythmias	Tachyarrythmias, hypertension

receptors are more abundant in coronary arterioles than in any other vascular area (6). A_1 and A_3 receptors also have a potential role in mediating preconditioning (6).

Adenosine is produced intracellularly via two pathways, but it does not exert its effects until it leaves the intracellular environment and it interacts with A_1 and A_2 adenosine receptors on the cell membrane (7). Dipyridamole acts by blocking the uptake and transport of adenosine into the cells, thereby resulting in a greater availability of adenosine at the receptor site. Both these mechanisms can provoke myocardial ischemia in the presence of a fixed reduction in coronary flow reserve due to epicardial coronary artery stenosis (7).

A. Mechanism of Supply–Demand Mismatch: Increase in Oxygen Demand

This mechanism can be easily fitted into the familiar concept framework of ischemia as a supply–demand mismatch, deriving from an increase in oxygen requirements in the presence of a fixed reduction in coronary flow reserve (Fig. 3). The different stresses can determine increases in demand through different mechanisms.

In resting conditions, myocardial oxygen consumption is dependent mainly upon heart rate, inotropic state, and the left ventricular wall stress (which is proportional to the systolic blood pressure) (8). Following dipyridamole or adenosine administration, a slight increase in myocardial function, a modest decrease in blood pressure, and mild tachycardia can be observed, overall determining only a trivial increase in myocardial oxygen demand (9).

During exercise, the increase in heart rate, blood pressure, and inotropic state accounts for the overall increase in myocardial oxygen consumption (Fig. 3). Pacing and dobutamine also increase—to a lesser degree—myocardial oxygen demand (9). During pacing, the increase is mainly due to the increased heart

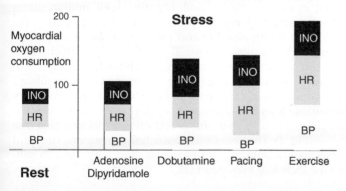

FIGURE 3 Major determinants of myocardial oxygen consumption in resting conditions (*left*) and during some stresses (*right*) commonly employed with echocardiography. The relative contributions of systolic blood pressure, heart rate, and inotropic state to myocardial oxygen demand are represented. During dipyridamole or adenosine stress, there is a mild increase in oxygen consumption for the increase in the inotropic state or heart rate, respectively. The rise in oxygen demand is even more marked during exercise, which causes an increase in heart rate as well as in inotropic state and systolic pressure. *Abbreviations*: INO, inotropic state; HR, heart rate; BP, systolic blood pressure. *Source*: From Ref. 8.

rate. Dobutamine markedly increases contractility and heart rate (Fig. 3). Further augment in myocardial oxygen consumption for heart rate increase occurs with the coadministration of atropine with dobutamine and dipyridamole.

B. Mechanism of Supply–Demand Mismatch: Reduction in Subendocardial Flow Supply

In the presence of coronary atherosclerosis, appropriate arteriolar dilation can paradoxically exert detrimental effects on regional myocardial perfusion, causing overperfusion of myocardial layers or regions already well perfused in resting conditions at the expense of regions or layers with a precarious flow balance in resting conditions (7). In "vertical steal," the anatomical requisite is the presence of an epicardial coronary artery stenosis and the subepicardium "steals" blood from the subendocardial layers. "Horizontal steal" requires the presence of collateral circulation between two vascular beds: the victim of the steal is the myocardium fed by the more stenotic vessel. The arteriolar vasodilatory reserve must be preserved—at least partially—in the donor vessel and abolished in the vessel receiving collateral flow (7). After vasodilation, the flow in the collateral circulation is reduced relative to resting conditions, since the arteriolar bed of the donor vessel "competes" with the arteriolar bed of the receiving vessel, whose vasodilatory reserve was already exhausted in resting conditions. The stresses provoking this flow maldistribution act through a "reverse Robin-Hood effect" (10); unlike the British hero who stole from the rich to give to the poor, they steal from the poor (myocardial regions or layers dependent upon a critically stenosed coronary artery) and give to the rich (regions or layers already well nourished in resting conditions). The biochemical effector of this hemodynamic mechanism is the inappropriate accumulation of adenosine, which is the main physiological modulator of coronary arteriolar vasodilation.

III. CORONARY FLOW RESERVE

In patients with normal coronary arteries and negative wall motion stress echocardiography, the assessment of coronary flow reserve by pulsed wave Doppler in mid-distal LAD is highly feasible and provides a simple and accurate assessment of coronary flow reserve (loops 27, 28, 81d, 83g), which has a strong prognostic power in several subsets of patients characterized by coronary microcirculatory involvement, from diabetes to hypertensives, from dilated to hypertrophic cardiomyopathy and chest pain patients with normal coronary arteries (11). The most suitable tests to assess coronary flow reserve are vasodilators, which at adequate doses can also be useful to test myocardial ischemia due to coronary artery disease (Fig. 4). They evoke a substantially greater recruitment of coronary flow reserve than dobutamine and exercise, and they are also substantially simpler from the technical viewpoint (12).

IV. STRESS ECHO FOR MYOCARDIAL VIABILITY

Asynergic, but viable, myocardium preserves a contractile reserve, which may be evoked by an appropriate stimulus (the kiss of the Prince Charming) awakening the seemingly dead myocardium (the sleeping beauty). The kiss may take place through a primary inotropic stimulus (determining a secondary increase in flow to meet the augmented metabolic demands) or through a primary metabolic stimulus (determining the increment in regional function) (13,14). The prototype

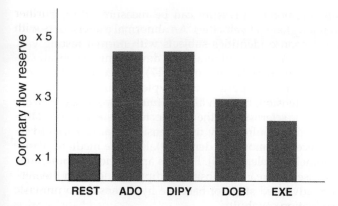

FIGURE 4 Coronary flow reserve and stresses. Vasodilators [adenosine (ADO) or dipyridamole (DIPY)] evoke a greater recruitment of coronary flow reserve, substantially higher than dobutamine (DOB) and exercise (EXE). They are more appropriate stressors for testing coronary flow reserve. *Source*: From Ref. 11.

of an inotropic stress for viability assessment is low-dose dobutamine, but similar results can be obtained with other inotropic (enoximone) or vasodilatory (dipyridamole, adenosine, nitrates) stimuli (loops 44–50). The possibility of recruiting a coronary flow reserve might appear paradoxical in the presence of resting dysfunction due to stunning or hibernation. The traditional concept is that a decrease in resting coronary blood flow indicates that coronary vasodilating reserve was fully exhausted. However, viable segments do have some vasodilatory reserve, which is mirrored by contractile reserve (15), possibly a last line of defence to cope with life-threatening situations with increased adrenergic drive putting the heart at risk for acute left ventricular failure.

V. STRESS ECHO IN VALVULAR HEART DISEASE

In valvular heart disease such as symptomatic mild mitral stenosis or mild-to-moderate aortic stenosis with depressed left ventricular function, stress echo can be useful to assess dynamically the disease severity with functional testing. The increase in cardiac output and transvalvular flow can be achieved with exercise or dobutamine (loops 70a–b). This will disproportionately increase the transvalvular gradient only when the valve area is severely reduced. Some patients with low gradient aortic stenosis have a low calculated aortic valve area because there is not enough forward flow to open the valve. In these patients, aortic valve area is not fixed but flow-dependent. Patients with "fixed severe stenosis" are likely to respond favorably to surgery (16). Patients with "pseudostenosis" have an increment in stroke volume with an increase in valve area and little change in gradient, suggesting that baseline evaluation overestimated the severity of stenosis (see Chap. 9).

VI. STRESS ECHO IN PULMONARY HYPERTENSION

In the development of pulmonary hypertension, there is a long preclinical stage characterized by normal resting values of systolic pulmonary pressure and increased reactivity of pulmonary microcirculation to vasoconstrictive stimuli such as exercise. Systolic pulmonary pressure can be measured during exercise from peak tricuspid regurgitant jet velocities. An abnormal exercise-induced pulmonary hypertensive response identifies subjects with normal resting values of pulmonary systolic pressure but vulnerable to developing genetically or environmentally mediated pulmonary hypertension (17). The genetically determined predisposition to pulmonary hypertension is typically observed not only in primary pulmonary hypertension, but can also be found in association with other diseases such as systemic sclerosis or other connective tissue diseases (18). The environmentally determined pulmonary hypertension is also observed in high-altitude or apnea-induced pulmonary edema (19). Exercise mediates vasoconstriction through endothelin-1 release (20). For this application, dobutamine is not a surrogate for exercise, whereas adenosine or dipyridamole can theoretically be useful at a more advanced stage of baseline hypertension to unmask residual pulmonary vasodilation capability.

DVD note: The following loops are related to the content of this chapter: 1–33, 44–50, 70a–b, 81d, 83g. These loops can be found in the provided DVD.

REFERENCES

1. Picano E. Stress Echocardiography, 4th ed. Heidelberg, Germany: Springer-Verlag, 2003.
2. Maseri A. Role of coronary artery spasm in symptomatic and silent myocardial ischemia. J Am Coll Cardiol 1987; 9:249–262.
3. Picano E, Mathias W Jr, Pingitore A, et al. On behalf of the EDIC Study Group, Safety and tolerability of dobutamine–atropine stress echocardiography: A prospective, large scale, multicenter trial. Lancet 1994; 344:1190–1192.
4. Picano E, Lattanzi F, Masini M, et al. Aminophylline termination of dipyridamole stress as a trigger of coronary vasospasm in variant angina. Am J Cardiol 1988; 62:694–697.
5. Ruffolo RR Jr, Spradlin TA, Pollock GD, et al. Alpha and beta adrenergic effects of the stereoisomers of dobutamine. J Pharmacol Exp Ther 1981; 219:447–452.
6. Fredholm BB, Abbracchio MP, Burnstock G, et al. Nomenclature and classification of purinoceptors. Pharmacol Rev 1994; 46:143–156.
7. Picano E. Dipyridamole-echocardiography test: Historical background and physiologic basis. Eur Heart J 1989; 10:365–376.
8. Ross J Jr. Factors regulating the oxygen consumption of the heart. In: Russek HI, Zoham BL, eds. Changing concepts in cardiovascular disease. Baltimore, MD: William & Wilkins, 1972:20–31.
9. Picano E. Stress echocardiography: From pathophysiological toy to diagnostic tool. Point of view. Circulation 1992; 85:1604–1612.
10. Picano E, Lattanzi F. Dipyridamole echocardiography: A new diagnostic window on coronary artery disease. Circulation 1991; 83(Suppl.):III19–III26.
11. Iskandrian AS, Verani MS, Heo J. Pharmacologic stress testing: Mechanism of action, hemodynamic responses, and results in detection of coronary artery disease. J Nucl Cardiol 1994; 1:94–111.
12. Rigo F. Coronary flow reserve in stress-echo lab. From pathophysiologic toy to diagnostic tool. Cardiovasc Ultrasound 2005; 3:8.
13. Pierard LA, De Landsheere CM, Berthe C, et al. Identification of viable myocardium by echocardiography during dobutamine infusion in patients with myocardial infarction after thrombolytic therapy: Comparison with positron emission tomography. J Am Coll Cardiol 1990; 15:1021–1031.

14. Picano E, Marzullo P, Gigli G, et al. Identification of viable myocardium by dipyridamole-induced improvement in regional left ventricular function assessed by echocardiography in myocardial infarction and comparison with thallium scintigraphy at rest. Am J Cardiol 1992; 70:703–710.
15. Torres MA, Picano E, Parodi G, et al. Flow-function relation in patients with chronic coronary artery disease and reduced regional function. A positron emission tomographic and two-dimensional echocardiographic study with coronary vasodilator stress. J Am Coll Cardiol 1997; 30:65–70.
16. Grayburn PA. Assessment of low-gradient aortic stenosis with dobutamine. Circulation 2006; 113:604–606.
17. Grunig E, Janssen B, Mereles D, et al. Abnormal pulmonary artery pressure response in asymptomatic carriers of primary pulmonary hypertension gene. Circulation 2000; 102:1145–1150.
18. Pignone A, Mori F, Pieri F, et al. Exercise Doppler echocardiography identifies preclinic asymptomatic pulmonary hypertension in systemic sclerosis. Ann N Y Acad Sci 2007; 1108:291–304.
19. Grunig E, Mereles D, Hildebrandt W, et al. Stress Doppler echocardiography for identification of susceptibility to high altitude pulmonary edema. J Am Coll Cardiol 2000; 35:980–987.
20. Sartori C, Allemann Y, Scherrer U. Pathogenesis of pulmonary edema: Learning from high-altitude pulmonary edema. Respir Physiol Neurobiol 2007; 159:338–349.

3 Environment, Facilities, Staff, Accreditation

Bogdan A. Popescu

"Carol Davila" University of Medicine and Pharmacy, and "C. C. Iliescu" Institute of Cardiovascular Diseases, Bucharest, Romania

Stress echocardiography has become a valuable method for cardiovascular stress testing and its clinical indications are currently extending beyond diagnostic assessment and risk stratification in patients with ischemic heart disease. Just like any other medical "tool," stress echocardiography performance should also meet quality standards in order to provide reliable information for clinical decision making. Efforts are being made by European and American Societies to elaborate recommendations in this regard.

I. ENVIRONMENT

Properly trained staff and appropriate equipment, placed in a designated room, large enough (e.g., >20 m^2) to accommodate all the facilities required for stress echocardiography testing and to allow sufficient patient and operator comfort (1), are "minimal" requirements for high-quality stress echo performance. Adequate ventilation, lighting, and heating should be in place. Echo machines generate heat, and in the absence of appropriate ventilation there is a risk of making the patients and the operator very uncomfortable, and shortening the lifespan of the machine (1).

Patient comfort, privacy, dignity, and provision of appropriate and clear information about the procedures must be considered (1). There must also be awareness of safety issues. A report database with facilities for storing and retrieving echo studies should exist. A viewing room, separate from the one used for patient' scanning, is recommended for review of studies and off-line reporting (1).

II. FACILITIES

Equipment requirements for a stress echocardiography laboratory are presented in Table 1. Good image quality is a "must" for stress echocardiography. Ultrasound systems must be equipped with stress echocardiography software, with minimal frame rate >40 frames/sec, digital acquisition with ECG triggering, and capacity for comprehensive imaging (1). As analyses of wall motion abnormalities continues to be the goal of most stress echo tests currently performed, tissue harmonic imaging is mandatory and should always be used as it reduces near-field artifact, improves resolution, enhances myocardial signals, and is superior to fundamental imaging for endocardial border detection (2,3). The improvement in endocardial visualization achieved with harmonic imaging has significantly decreased interobserver variability and has improved the sensitivity of stress echocardiography for the diagnosis of coronary artery disease (3–5).

TABLE 1   Equipment Requirements for a Stress Echocardiography Laboratory

---

Ultrasound systems provided with stress echocardiography software
Contrast agents and contrast specific software
Exercise/pharmacologic/electric stress facilities
   Exercise stress equipment: treadmill, sitting bicycle, supine bicycle, supine bicycle (tilted)
   Pharmacologic stressors: dobutamine, dipyridamole, adenosine, ergonovine, and their
      antidotes (β-blocker for dobutamine, aminophylline for dipyridamole, nitroglycerine for
      ergonovine)
   Transesophageal pacing and recording catheter (optional)
Ancillary facilities
   Examination table next to the treadmill
   Infusion syringe for pharmacological stress/contrast agents
   ECG monitor and recorder
   Sphygmomanometer
   Resuscitation apparatus and drugs
   Oxygen source

Use of digital frame grabbers and split or "quadscreen" displays allows side-by-side comparison of rest and stress images and is the current standard for the performance of stress echocardiograms (6). However, digital image acquisition and transfer to a computer workstation for off-line analysis is preferred, if possible, as review of multiple cardiac cycles with stress maximizes accuracy of interpretation (3). Videotape recordings are currently recommended only as a backup (3). Echo machines should be serviced regularly.

Provision of additional hardware and software for improving quantification (contrast agents and contrast specific software or tissue Doppler) is desirable and should ideally be available (1). When used in conjunction with harmonic imaging, contrast agents increase the number of interpretable left ventricular wall segments, improve the accuracy of less-experienced readers, enhance diagnostic confidence, and reduce the need for additional noninvasive tests required because of equivocal noncontrast stress examinations (3,7–10). With experience and well-defined protocols, contrast stress echocardiography has been shown to be time-efficient (11).

Both treadmill and bicycle exercise systems should be available in any stress echo laboratory, as exercise stress testing is preferred and recommended in all patients who are capable to exercise according to their ability to perform a certain type of effort (e.g., walking or pedaling). When stress echocardiography is combined with treadmill exercise, the images are acquired right before starting the test and immediately after the occurrence of the exercise-limiting symptoms (preferably within 60–90 seconds after exercise termination, as ischemia-induced wall motion abnormalities may resolve quickly postexercise). With appropriate training and expertise, success rates higher than 95% should be attained (6).

Bicycle stress echocardiography can be performed with either supine or upright ergometry and has the advantage of allowing imaging at incremental levels of stress including peak exercise. Supine and upright bicycle exercises appear to have equivalent degrees of accuracy (6). Supine bicycle ergometry has the specific advantage of allowing Doppler interrogation of mitral, tricuspid, and aortic-valve flows during exercise. For centers using a bicycle ergometer, rotation up to a 45° angle should be available, having the possibility to position the patient in a 45° angle backwards, and a 45° angle rotated to the left side (1).

Different pharmacological stressors, such as dobutamine and vasodilators (dypiridamole, adenosine) should be available as they are necessary in patients who cannot exercise.

Transesophageal atrial pacing stress echocardiography is another option for the detection of coronary artery disease in patients unable to exercise (12). It requires a pacing catheter (housed in a 10F sheath) that may be placed orally or nasally after topical anesthesia and advanced by having the patient swallow while in the left lateral decubitus position. The advantage of pacing is the rapid restoration of baseline conditions and heart rate on discontinuation of the atrial stimulus; this avoids a prolonged state of ischemia (13). Side effects, except for mild atrial arrhythmogenicity, are uncommon. Although it is not commonly used, transesophageal atrial pacing is an effective and safe modality for inducing ischemia (14).

Infusion syringe for pharmacological stress, an ECG monitor and recorder, as well as sphygmomanometer and oxygen source are mandatory equipments in a stress echocardiography laboratory. Resuscitation apparatus and drugs must be readily available (1).

III. STAFF

Stress echocardiography is one of the most demanding echocardiographic techniques requiring appropriate skills both in acquiring good-quality images during stress and in interpretation of these images. It is therefore not reasonable to start doing stress echocardiography without full training in transthoracic echocardiography (TTE). On the other hand, stressing the patient and inducing myocardial ischaemia carries a distinct risk of complications and requires the ability to safely monitor stress in a person with potentially severe cardiovascular disease. For all these reasons, the examination should be performed only in laboratories staffed by trained personnel on appropriately monitored patients. The personnel requirements and the level of monitoring required will vary with local standards of care and the type of stress being employed (15) (Table 2).

At least two persons are required to record and monitor stress echocardiography studies. If the study is not performed by a physician but by a sonographer/technician, a physician with expertise in both echocardiography and resuscitation should be available in the immediate vicinity in case an acute problem occurs. One of the personnel present should be qualified in advanced life support, the other in basic life support. Personnel should be sufficiently trained in contrast echocardiography when contrast is given; the possibility of hypersensitivity should be anticipated (15). Interpretation of stress echocardiograms requires extensive experience in echocardiography and should be performed only by physicians with specific training in the technique (6). The American Society of Echocardiography recommendations for performance, interpretation, and appliance of stress echocardiography (2003) state that only echocardiographers with at least Level 2 of echo training and with specific additional training in stress echocardiography may have the responsibility for supervision and interpretation of stress echocardiograms (6). In addition to Level 2 training, supervised overreading of at least 100 stress echocardiograms under the supervision of an echocardiographer with level 3 training and expertise in stress echocardiography is required to attain the minimum level of competence for independent interpretation (14). To maintain competence it is recommended that physicians interpret

TABLE 2 Staff Requirements for a Stress Echocardiography Laboratory

- At least two persons are required to record and monitor stress echo studies
- One of the personnel present should be qualified in Advanced Life Support, the other in Basic Life Support
- If the study is performed by a sonographer/technician, a physician with expertise in both echocardiography and resuscitation should be available in the immediate vicinity in case an acute problem occurs

Training requirements for the performance and interpretation of stress echocardiography, according to ACC/AHA clinical competence statement on echocardiography (14):

- Understanding of the basic principles, indications, applications, and technical limitations of echocardiography.
- Level 2 training in transthoracic echocardiography.
- Specialized training in stress echocardiography with performance and interpretation of ≥100 stress studies under appropriate supervision by a Level 3 echocardiographer.

Maintenance of competence in stress echocardiography (14):

- Performance and interpretation of at least 100 stress studies per year.
- Participation in continuing medical education in echocardiography (minimum of 5 hr/yr of CME credits in echocardiography, as recommended by the Intersocietal Commission for the Accreditation of Echocardiography Laboratories, ICAEL) (18)
- Proof-of-competence and maintenance of competence recommendations for contrast echocardiography have not been established. For now, it is accepted that physicians with Level 2 competence in echocardiography who have learned how to apply contrast agents and interpret contrast-enhanced studies are competent (14).

a minimum of 100 stress echocardiograms per year, in addition to participating in relevant continuing medical education activities (16). It is recommended that sonographers perform a minimum of 100 stress echocardiograms per year to maintain an appropriate level of skill (16). These recommendations refer to routine stress echocardiograms for evaluation of coronary artery disease and do not apply for highly specialized studies such as evaluation of valvular heart disease or myocardial viability, for which more experience and higher volumes may be required for skills maintenance (3).

IV. ACCREDITATION

For proper and safe performance of stress echocardiography, accreditation of both the individual performing the study and the laboratory where the study is performed should be mandatory. Establishing clear standards for the requirements of personnel training, staffing level, and equipment available in a stress echo laboratory is an important measure with the ultimate goal of safeguarding patients undergoing stress echocariograms.

For performing and interpreting stress echocardiograms, the physician should have enough expertise in TTE; in European countries, the European Association of Echocardiography (EAE) individual accreditation or the national accreditation in TTE should be a prerequisite before starting stress echocardiography. The EAE accreditation in TTE, started in 2003, can be obtained after passing a written examination (held twice a year) consisting of a Theory section (100 multiple choice questions) and a Reporting section (50 multiple choice questions based on 10 cases covering a wide range of pathology). Candidates who have passed the exam need then to submit, within 1 year from the written exam, a logbook of 250 cases performed and reported by themselves, which will be assessed by expert external reviewers (17). Those who also pass the logbook receive the EAE accreditation diploma, which is valid for 5 years, after which reaccreditation becomes necessary (17). So far, no individual accreditation system specifically designed for stress echocardiography exists at the European level.

In the EAE recommendations for laboratory standards and accreditation (1), a module specifically designed for stress echocardiography performance is described. There should be a designated Head of Stress Echocardiography, directly involved in stress echoes and reporting at least 100 stress echocardiograms annually. A detailed specific request form including indications for stress, clinical data, medications, allergies, and other relevant details (e.g., history of asthma, prostatism, glaucoma) should be listed (1).

Any operator who reports stress echocardiograms must be specifically trained in stress echocardiography and be authorized by the Head of Stress Echo. A list of indications for stress echocardiograms should be agreed, appropriate protocols for studies (including acquisition and display details) should be established and all the operators in the laboratory must adhere to them.

Quality control should be ensured by means of regular audits, by regular (e.g., weekly) meetings of the staff involved in stress echo, and by comparison of stress echo results with other techniques, including (but not limited to) coronary angiography (1).

In order to reach the advanced standards, scientific work, research, and publications will be considered. For the stress echo laboratory to qualify for the advanced level, at least 300 stress echo studies should be performed yearly in the lab, using more than one modality (pharmacological and exercise) (1). The number of staff personnel and work-hours must be adequate for the number of in-training people, in order to assure appropriate training. There should be access to local, national, and international meetings for the staff involved in stress echocardiography. There should also be free access to paper and online journals for all staff. A core library with updated echocardiography and cardiology textbooks, as well as training materials (tapes, CDs, electronic cases, etc.), and internet access should be available to all staff (1).

Stress echocardiography has a great potential for diagnostic, prognostic, and therapeutic purposes. However, this statement is true only if stress echocardiograms are performed appropriately by a well-trained staff, on adequately equipped machines, in a specifically designed laboratory, with careful monitoring. Otherwise, performance of stress echocardiography should be avoided, as it may turn into a dangerous adventure.

REFERENCES

1. Nihoyannopoulos P, Fox K, Fraser A, et al.; On behalf of the Laboratory Accreditation Committee of the European Association of Echocardiography. EAE laboratory standards and accreditation. Eur J Echocardiogr 2007; 8:80–87.
2. Skolnick D, Sawada S, Feigenbaum H, et al. Enhanced endocardial visualization with noncontrast harmonic imaging during stress echocardiography. J Am Soc Echocardiogr 1999; 12:559–563.
3. Pellikka PA, Nagueh SF, Elhendy AA, et al. American society of echocardiography recommendations for performance, interpretation, and application of stress echocardiography. J Am Soc Echocardiogr 2007; 9:1021–1041.

4. Franke A, Hoffman R, Kuhl H. Non-contrast second harmonic imaging improves interobserver agreement and accuracy of dobutamine stress echocardiography in patients with impaired image quality. Heart 2000; 83:133–140.
5. Sozi F, Poldermans D, Bax J. Second harmonic imaging improves sensitivity of dobutamine stress echocardiography for the diagnosis of coronary artery disease. Am Heart J 2001; 142:153–159.
6. Armstrong WF, Pellikka PA, Ryan T, et al. Stress echocardiography: Recommendations for performance and interpretation of stress echocardiography. Stress Echocardiography Task Force of the Nomenclature and Standards Committee of the American Society of Echocardiography. J Am Soc Echocardiogr 1998; 11:97–104.
7. Rainbird A, Mulvagh S, Oh J, et al. Contrast dobutamine stress echocardiography: Clinical practice assessment in 300 consecutive patients. J Am Soc Echocardiogr 2001; 14:378–385.
8. Vlassak I, Rubin D, Odabashian J. Contrast and harmonic imaging improves the accuracy and efficiency of novice readers for dobutamine stress echocardiography. Echocardiography 2002; 19:483–488.
9. Dolan M, Riad K, El-Shafei A. Effect of intravenous contrast for left ventricular opacification and border definition on sensitivity and specificity of dobutamine stress echocardiography compared with coronary angiography in technically difficult patients. Am Heart J 2001; 142:908–915.
10. Thanigaraji S, Nease R, Schechtman K, et al. Use of contrast for image enhancement during stress echocardiography is cost-effective and reduces additional diagnostic testing. Am J Cardiol 2001; 87:1430–1432.
11. Castello R, Bella J, Rovner A, et al. Efficacy and time-efficiency of "sonographer-driven" contrast echocardiography protocol in a high-volume echocardiography laboratory. Am Heart J 2003; 145:535–541.
12. Lee C, Pellikka P, McCully R, et al. Non-exercise stress transthoracic echocardiography: Transesophageal atrial pacing versus dobutamine stress. J Am Coll Cardiol 1999; 33:506–511.
13. Rainbird A, Pellikka P, Stussy V, et al. A rapid stress-testing protocol for the detection of coronary artery disease: Comparison of two-stage transesophageal atrial pacing stress echocardiography with dobutamine stress echocardiography. J Am Coll Cardiol 2000; 36:1659–1663.
14. Quinones M, Douglas P, Foster E, et al. ACC/AHA clinical competence statement on echocardiography: A report of the American College of Cardiology/American Heart Association/American College of Physicians-American Society of Internal Medicine task force on clinical competence. J Am Coll Cardiol 2003; 41:687–708.
15. Becher H, Chambers J, Fox K, et al. BSE procedure guidelines for the clinical application of stress echocardiography, recommendations for performance and interpretation of stress echocardiography: A report of the British Society of Echocardiography Policy Committee. Heart 2004; 90:23–30.
16. Bierig S, Ehler D, Knoll M, et al. American Society of Echocardiography minimum standards for the cardiac sonographer: A position paper. J Am Soc Echocardiogr 2006; 19:471–474.
17. www.escardio.org/bodies/associations/EAE/accreditation/TTE.
18. ICAEL Newsletter 2001, vol. 4; Issue 2; p. 5.

Stress Echocardiography Examination: Imaging, Reading, and Quantification

Rosa Sicari

CNR, Institute of Clinical Physiology, Pisa, Italy

I. GENERAL TEST PROTOCOL

The patient lies in lateral decubitus, the position required to achieve an optimal echocardiographic view. Electrocardiographic leads are placed at standard limb and precordial sites, slightly displacing (upward and downward) any leads that may interfere with the chosen acoustic windows. A 12-lead echocardiography is recorded in resting condition and each minute throughout the examination. An echocardiography lead is also continuously displayed on the echo monitor to provide the operator with a reference for ST-segment changes and arrhythmias. Cuff blood pressure is measured in resting condition and each stage thereafter. Echocardiographic imaging is typically performed from the parasternal long- and short-axis, apical long-axis, and apical four- and two-chamber views. In some cases the subxyphoidal and apical long-axis views are used. Images are recorded in resting condition from all views and captured digitally. A quad-screen format is used for comparative analysis. Recording on videotape alone is not sufficient and may be used as a backup medium only in cases of technical failure (1).

Echocardiography is then continuously monitored and intermittently stored. In the presence of obvious or suspected dyssynergy, a complete echo examination is performed and recorded from all employed approaches to allow optimal documentation of the presence and extent of myocardial ischemia. These same projections are obtained and recorded during the recovery phase, after cessation of stress (exercise or pacing) or administration of the antidote (amino-phylline for dipyridamole, β-blocker for dobutamine, and nitroglycerine for ergometrine) (1); an ischemic response may occasionally occur late, after cessation of drug infusion (2). In this way, the transiently dyssynergic area during stress can be evaluated by a triple comparison: stress versus resting state, stress versus recovery phase, and at peak stress. It is critical to obtain the same views at each stage of the test. Analysis and scoring of the study are usually performed using a 16- or 17-segment model of the left ventricle (1–3) and a four-grade scale of regional wall motion analysis. Diagnostic end points of stress echocardiographic testing are maximum dose (for pharmacological) or maximum workload (for exercise testing), achievement of target heart rate, obvious echocardiographic positivity (with akinesis of ≥2 left ventricular segments), severe chest pain, or obvious electrocardiographic positivity (with >2 mV ST-segment shift). Submaximal nondiagnostic end points of stress echo testing are nontolerable symptoms or limiting asymptomatic side effects such as hypertension, with systolic blood pressure >220 mm Hg or diastolic blood pressure >120 mm Hg;

symptomatic hypotension, with >40 mm Hg drop in blood pressure; supraventricular arrhythmias, such as supraventricular tachycardia or atrial fibrillations; and complex ventricular arrhythmias, such as ventricular tachycardia or frequent, polymorphic premature ventricular beats.

There are a few general rules that can be followed in setting up a stress echo laboratory: The choice of one test over the other depends on patient characteristics, local drug cost, and the physician's preference. It is important for all stress echocardiography laboratories to become familiar with all stresses to achieve a flexible and versatile diagnostic approach that enables the best stress to be tailored to individual patient needs. Physical or pharmacological (inotropic or vasodilator) stress echocardiography has comparable diagnostic accuracies. The choice of one test over the other will depend on relative contraindications. Large-volume laboratories should be fully acquainted with all the three main forms of stress in order to apply the test in all patients. In the presence of a submaximal first-line stress for limiting side effects, the second choice should be applied, since submaximal (physical or pharmacological) stresses have suboptimal diagnostic value. The less informative and/or interpretable exercise electrocardiography is, the higher the level of appropriateness to stress echocardiography. Both dobutamine and dipyridamole should be performed with high-dose protocols to obtain high sensitivities, comparable to maximal exercise. The standard protocols and the addition of atropine should be followed in order to obtain the target heart rate (especially for dobutamine stress echocardiography). Handgrip is an acceptable alternative to atropine in case of contraindications.

II. STRESS ECHOCARDIOGRAPHY: TECHNOLOGY AND TRAINING

A few simple recommendations regarding the apparatus, the stresses, and the echocardiographer can help to move stress echocardiography from scientific journals to the reader's laboratory.

A. The Machine

The Doppler (pulsed, continuous, and color-coded) is an "optional" in stress echocardiography, while good quality of the echocardiographic image is absolutely necessary. Poor image quality will imply a larger number of patients with a technically not suitable baseline visualization and a higher percentage of patients in whom the suboptimal visualization of the endocardium will make wall motion evaluation "uncertain" or "questionable." Refinement of image technology will increase the overall feasibility of stress echocardiography, improve diagnostic performance, and deflate interobserver variability. A good 2-D echocardiographic machine is not a surrogate for an adequate training of the cardiologist, but it gives the experienced operator the opportunity to exploit the potentials of stress echocardiography to the fullest.

Digital Acquisition

By digitizing the 2-D echocardiographic images, it is possible to place a single cardiac cycle into a continuous loop so that the cycle can be viewed whenever necessary for an indefinite period of time. This technique carries valuable advantages, especially for exercise echocardiography (1). Even in the exercising individual who is breathing rapidly and deeply, one can still see a technically good cardiac cycle between inspirations; therefore, it reduces the respiratory artifact.

Another advantage of using the computer to record the 2-D echocardiogram digitally is that it is possible to place the resting and stress cardiac cycles side by side in a split-screen or quad-screen format. This reduces the time and difficulty of analyzing the examination and may also simplify the recognition of subtle changes in wall motion. Digital storage and review is now the state of the art in echocardiography. Although secondary digitization from videotape may be an acceptable transitional solution, the ultimate benefits of the digital laboratory can only be achieved with direct digital output from a contemporary echocardiography machine (4). This is particularly true with the current generation of echo instruments that have the option for digital acquisition in the software, with the possibility of digitizing the recordings both off-line from videotape and on-line during the actual examinations. Digital acquisition has further boosted the spread of the stress echocardiography technique, reducing the time needed for and the difficulty inherent in image acquisition and interpretation. Although there is no evidence showing that it improves diagnostic accuracy when compared with videotape reading, digital acquisition certainly makes storage, retrieval, analysis, and communication of stress echocardiography data faster and easier (5).

Tissue Harmonic Imaging

Tissue harmonic imaging should be used for stress echocardiography imaging (1). This reduces near-field artifact, improves resolution, enhances myocardial signals, and is superior to fundamental imaging for endocardial border visualization. The increased image quality is mirrored in a better visualization of the left ventricular endocardium and myocardium. In the stress echocardiography setting, tissue harmonic imaging reduces the number of uninterpretable segments, reduces observer variability, and increases diagnostic accuracy. The number of uninterpretable segments is reduced by approximately 30% to 50% with tissue harmonic imaging in the setting of stress echocardiography (6–10) and allows application of stress echocardiography to technically difficult patients previously deemed unsuitable for this test. The increase in interpretable myocardium is particularly valuable for the apical, lateral, and anterior wall segments imaged in the apical views (6,7) at higher heart rates (11). Tissue harmonic imaging reduces interobserver variability for wall motion assessment among expert readers (6,7). This is a direct consequence of the improved quality of the echocardiographic images (12). On the other hand, improved image quality by tissue harmonic imaging seems not to improve diagnostic accuracy of experienced observers (8), supporting the general rule that it is better to have experienced eyes with suboptimal technology than advanced technology with inexperienced eyes.

B. The Echocardiographer

Prerequisites

It is not reasonable to begin using stress echocardiography without a complete training in transthoracic echocardiography. The basic skills required for imaging the heart under resting conditions are not substantially different from those required for imaging the same heart from the same projections during stress. Furthermore, the echocardiographic signs of ischemia are basically the same as those during myocardial infarction. One might even say that the diagnosis of transient ischemia can be easier than the diagnosis of infarction. In both cases, the assessment is based upon a comparison between the "suspected" zone and the neighboring normal regions; in induced ischemia, however, the operator can use the suspected region as its own control, considering both resting conditions and the recovery phase.

The setting up of a stress echo laboratory requires dedicated personnel and equipment. A registered nurse with Basic Life Support and Advanced Cardiac Life Support training will attend each single examination, prepare the patients, the drugs to be infused, and check clinical status, heart rate, blood pressure, and ECG. A physician will always attend the examination, eventually as it is standard procedure in Europe, scan, store and analyze images, and prepare the final report. The laboratory will be equipped with resuscitation equipment (defibrillator, intubation kit, etc.) and all the standard necessary drugs should be available at hand in case of life-threatening complications. In summary, the stress echo laboratory should be run as any other facility dealing with potential major complications of myocardial ischemia. Moreover, the personnel consisting of at least two people (a nurse and a physician) should be familiar with all the potential complications of stressors employed to induce myocardial ischemia.

Training and Interpretation

It is not reasonable to begin using stress echocardiography without a complete training in transthoracic echocardiography, and the EAE accreditation exam is highly recommended. Moreover, careful monitoring of vital signs (clinical status, heart rate, blood pressure, and ECG beyond echo) is required during stress echocardiography, which should be done by cardiologists with Basic Life Support and Advanced Cardiac Life Support training. The basic skills required for imaging the heart under resting conditions do not differ substantially from those required for imaging the same heart from the same projections during stress. The diagnostic accuracy of an experienced echocardiographer who is an absolute beginner in stress echocardiography is more or less equivalent to that achieved by tossing a coin. However, 100 stress echocardiographic studies are more than adequate to build the individual learning curve and reach the plateau of diagnostic accuracy (13) (Fig. 1). It is wise to do the following: start with low-dose tests for viability and later progress to tests for ischemia; start with safer and easier vasodilator tests and later progress to adrenergic stresses; and start with pharmacological and then progress to physical exercise stress echocardiography. In the case of a patient with a known or suspected infarction, no echocardiographer would make the diagnosis of presence, site, and extension of dyssynergy on the basis of a single cardiac cycle in one view from only one approach: the dyssynergy can be highly localized, and some regions can be adequately visualized only in some projections. An important general rule of stress echocardiography stems from an obvious fact: all views that can be obtained should be obtained both in resting conditions and during stress. It is also evident that the temporal sampling must be continuous so that the exact ischemia-free stress time can be determined and the stress immediately stopped as soon as an obvious dyssynergy develops. Today, the interpretation of stress echocardiography is by necessity qualitative and subjective. Diagnostic accuracy is not only a function of experience; for a given diagnostic accuracy every observer has his/her own sensitivity–specificity

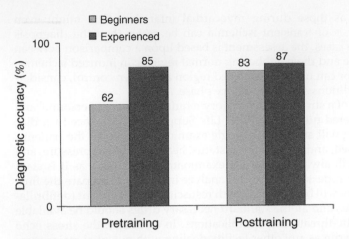

FIGURE 1 Histograms showing the diagnostic accuracy of the five beginners (*black bars*) and five experts (*gray bars*) who reviewed two sets of 50 videotapes before and after 6 months (100 stress echocardiography studies with a supervisor) training period. *Source*: From Ref. 13.

curve: there are "overreaders" (high sensitivity, low specificity) and "underreaders" (low sensitivity, high specificity), depending on whether images are aggressively or conservatively interpreted as abnormal. Many studies are unquestionably negative or positive; still, there is a "gray zone" of interpretable tests in which the visualization of some regions can be suboptimal and the cardiologist's level of experience in interpreting the test is critical for a correct reading (Figs. 2–4). Interobserver variability is certainly a common problem in medicine, and in cardiology variability can be substantial with almost all diagnostic methods, including resting electrocardiography (14), exercise electrocardiography (15), perfusion scintigraphy (16), and coronary angiography (17). There are many precautions that may minimize variability, providing not only high accuracy but also better reproducibility. These parameters are related to the physician interpreting the study, the technology used, the stress employed, and the patient

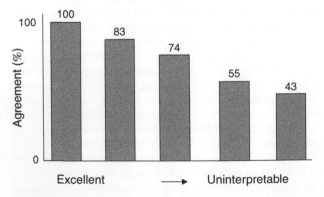

FIGURE 2 Factors modulating interpretation variability: image quality. Variability is substantially higher for poor-quality images.

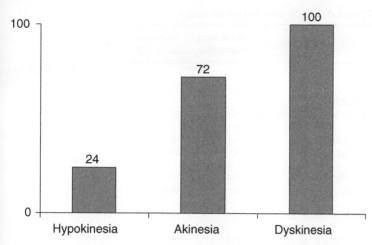

FIGURE 3 Factors modulating interpretation variability: severity of dysfunction. Variability is substantially higher for a mild degree of dysfunction such as hypokinesia.

under study (Tables 1–3). Variability will be substantially reduced if one agrees in advance not to consider minor degrees of hypokinesis, since mild hypokinesis is a normal variant under most stresses and finds a wide overlapping between a normal and a diseased population (18–21). The inclusion among positivity criteria of isolated asynergy of basal inferolateral or basal inferoseptal segments will also inflate variability. Obviously, the inclusion of patients with resting images of borderline quality or the use of stresses degrading image quality will also dilate variability, which is tightly linked to the quality of the images. Other factors including new technologies such as tissue Doppler have a potential

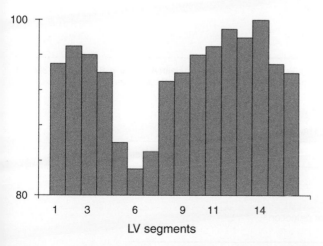

FIGURE 4 Factors modulating interpretation variability: location of wall motion abnormalities. Variability is substantially higher for tricky segments, such as basal inferolateral segment or basal inferior septum, which may be "physiologically hypokinetic" even at baseline.

TABLE 1 Stress Echocardiography and the Human Factor

	Increases variability	Decreases variability
Physician related		
Previous training in stress echo	No	Yes
Exposure to joint reading	No	Yes
Development of "a priori" reading criteria	No	Yes
Basal inferior septum	Yes	No
Positivity for "lack of hyperkinesis"	Yes	No
Positivity for "severe hypokinesis"	No	Yes
Technology related		
Videotape instead of digital	Yes	No
Native tissue harmonic	No	Yes
Stress related		
Use of stressor polluting image quality	Yes	No
Patient related		
Resting images of borderline quality	Yes	No

TABLE 2 Checklist to Start: The Human Factor; Training: Six Simple Necessary Rules

	To start	To learn	To keep competence	Top level
Certified competence in resting TTE (EAE)	√			
BLS and ACLS certification (AHA)	√			
Cardiology experience with exercise stress testing	√			
100 stresses with angiographic verification in a high-volume center		√		
100 stress echo per year			√	
Familiarity with all stressors (exercise, vasodilators, inotropic)				√
Mixed conditions (ischemia, valvular, cardiomyopathy)				√

Abbreviations: ACLS, advanced cardiac life support; AHA, American Heart Association; BLS, basic life support; EAE, European Association of Echocardiography; TTE, transthoracic echocardiography.

TABLE 3 Checklist to Start: The Technology Factor

	Helpful	Useless
Tissue harmonic imaging	√	
Digital	√	
Ergometer for exercise	√	
Intravenous contrast for border detection	√	
TDI, SRI, 3D, VVI		√

Abbreviations: SRI, strain rate imaging; TDI, tissue Doppler imaging; 3D, three-dimensional echocardiography.

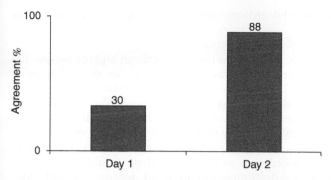

FIGURE 5 Bar histogram showing the class concordance in interpreting the studies at the beginning (day 1, pretraining) and at the end (day 2, posttraining) of the 2-day training session. There is a highly significant increase in the number of concordant interpretations. *Source*: From Ref. 25.

to reduce variability (22). Digital acquisition may improve reproducibility (20). In patients with a difficult acoustic window, native second harmonic imaging and the use of contrast agents help to improve accuracy and reduce variability (23,24). Finally, the single most important factor decreasing variability is a specific course of training in a large-volume stress echocardiography laboratory with exposure to joint reading (25) and "a priori" development of standardized (26) and conservative (27) reading criteria (Fig. 5).

C. Quantification

The objective operator-independent assessment of myocardial ischemia during stress echocardiography remains a technologic challenge. Still, adequate quality of two-dimensional images remains a prerequisite to successful quantitative analysis, even using Doppler-based techniques. No new technology has proved to have a higher diagnostic accuracy than conventional visual wall motion analysis (28). Tissue Doppler imaging (TDI) and derivatives may reduce interobserver variability, but still require a dedicated learning curve and special expertise. The development of contrast media in echocardiography has been slow. In the past decade, transpulmonary contrast agents have become commercially available for clinical use. The approved indication for the use of contrast echocardiography currently lies in improving endocardial border delineation in patients in whom adequate imaging is difficult or suboptimal (2). It is possible that these technologies may serve as an adjunct to expert visual assessment of wall motion. At present, these quantitative methods require further validation and simplification of analysis techniques (1,2).

III. FREQUENT MISTAKES ON STRESS ECHOCARDIOGRAPHY

A minimum of 100 supervised stress echocardiogram interpretations, in addition to advanced training in echocardiography, are recommended to cardiologists to establish competency in stress echocardiography (1,2,5). However, regardless of the number of stress echocardiography studies performed and intensity of training, some readers still do not reach a satisfactory accuracy (27). The six most frequent mistakes in stress echocardiography training can be summarized as follows:

1. *Self-made stress echocardiography*: It is far better to perform and/or review 100 stress echocardiography studies with an expert supervisor than 1000 stress echocardiography studies done all by yourself without a standard, a comparison, and a partner. Avoid self-taught stress echocardiography training!
2. *Start your learning curve from University*: Exercise is the most familiar stress to the cardiologist and the patient, but by far the most technically demanding.
3. *Use only one stressors*: A large-volume laboratory should be acquainted to all forms of stressors, in order to avoid potential contraindications (e.g., patients with a history of arrhythmias should avoid dobutamine and those with asthma should avoid dipyridamole).
4. *Underestimate the ischemic risk*: The technicalities of pharmacological stress echocardiography can be surprisingly simple, but one has to know how to treat ischemia and its unforeseeable and thrilling complications. A stress echocardiography laboratory run by technicians and sonographers can be a deadly trap for the patient.
5. *Skills in resting echo are not enough*: Pediatric, transesophageal, transthoracic, and vascular echo speak a different ultrasound idiom than stress echocardiography does. It is a different language and you have to learn it with dedicated training. It is not enough to have deep theoretical and experimental knowledge on regional wall motion determinants, you have to practice it in the clinical arena.
6. *Technology without cardiology*: It is better to have the best eyes with a suboptimal technology than the worst eyes with the best technology. Usually, there is economic interest in selling technology, not in the improvement of culture. However, sophisticated technology without know-how is blind, although know-how without appropriate machines can be hollow. Expensive products are not a surrogate of endogenous motivation! A crowded environment, doing several stresses per day, using with versatility all main forms of exercise, vasodilator, and adrenergic stresses, with different doctors rotating in the stress laboratory, with one nurse overstressed, and several patients waiting for their turn, it is probably the most appropriate way to perform stress echo.

REFERENCES

1. Pellikka PA, Nagueh SF, Elhendy AA, et al; American Society of Echocardiography. American Society of Echocardiography recommendations for performance, interpretation, and application of stress echocardiography. J Am Soc Echocardiogr 2007; 20:1021–1041.
2. Sicari R, Nihoyannopoulos P, Evangelista A, et al. Stress echocardiography expert consensus statement from the European association of echocardiography. Eur J Echocardiogr 2008; 9:415–437.
3. Cerqueira MD, Weissman NJ, Dilsizian V, et al; American Heart Association Writing Group on Myocardial Segmentation and Registration for Cardiac Imaging. Standardized myocardial segmentation and nomenclature for tomographic imaging of the heart: A statement for healthcare professionals from the Cardiac Imaging Committee of the Council on Clinical Cardiology of the American Heart Association. Circulation 2002; 105:539–542.

4. Thomas JD, Adams DB, Devries S, et al; Digital Echocardiography Committee of the American Society of Echocardiography. Guidelines and recommendations for digital echocardiography. J Am Soc Echocardiogr 2005; 18:287–297.
5. Nihoyannopoulos P, Fox K, Fraser A, et al; Laboratory Accreditation Committee of the EAE. EAE laboratory standards and accreditation. Eur J Echocardiogr 2007; 8:80–87.
6. Skolnick DG, Sawada SG, Feigenbaum H, et al. Enhanced endocardial visualization with noncontrast harmonic imaging during stress echocardiography. J Am Soc Echocardiogr 1999; 12:559–563.
7. Zaglavara T, Norton M, Cumberledge B, et al. Dobutamine stress echocardiography: Improved endocardial border definition and wall motion analysis with tissue harmonic imaging. J Am Soc Echocardiogr 1999; 12:706–713.
8. Rodriguez O, Varga A, Dal Porto R, et al. The impact of second harmonic imaging on stress echocardiography reading. Cardiologia 1999; 44:451–454.
9. Finkelhor RS, Pajouh M, Kett A, et al. Clinical impact of second harmonic imaging and left heart contrast in echocardiographic stress testing. Am J Cardiol 2000; 85:740–743.
10. Nixdorff U, Matschke C, Winklmaier M, et al. Native tissue second harmonic imaging improves endocardial and epicardial border definition in dobutamine stress echocardiography. Eur J Echocardiogr 2001; 2:52–61.
11. Sozzi FB, Poldermans D, Bo ersma E, et al. Does second harmonic imaging improve left ventricular endocardial border identification at higher heart rates during dobutamine stress echocardiography? J Am Soc Echocardiogr 2000; 13:1019–1024.
12. Hoffman R, Lethen H, Marwick TH, et al. Analysis of interinstitutional observer agreement in the interpretation of dobutamine stress-echocardiograms. J Am Coll Cardiol 1996; 27:330–336.
13. Picano E, Lattanzi F, Orlandini A, et al. Stress echocardiography and the human factor: The importance of being expert. J Am Coll Cardiol 1991; 17:666–669.
14. Segall HN. The electrocardiogram and its interpretation: A study of reports by 20 physicians on a set of 100 electrocardiograms. Can Med Assoc 1960; 82:2–6.
15. Blackburn H. The exercise electrocardiogram: Differences in interpretation. Am J Cardiol 1968; 21:871–880.
16. Atwood JE, Jensen D, Froelicher V, et al. Agreement in human interpretation of analog thallium myocardial perfusion images. Circulation 1981; 64:601–609.
17. Zir LM, Miller SW, Dinsmore RE, et al. Interobserver variability in coronary angiography. Circulation 1976; 53:627–632.
18. Borges AC, Pingitore A, Cordovil A, et al. Heterogeneity of left ventricular regional wall thickening following dobutamine infusion in normal human subjects. Eur Heart J 1995; 16:1726–1730.
19. Carstensen S, Ali SM, Stensgaard-Hansen FV, et al. Dobutamine-atropine stress echocardiography in asymptomatic healthy individuals. The relativity of stress-induced hyperkinesia. Circulation 1995; 92:3453–3463.
20. Castini D, Gentile F, Ornaghi M, et al. Dobutamine echocardiography: Usefulness of digital image processing. Eur Heart J 1995; 16:1420–1424.
21. Hoffmann R, Marwick TH, Poldermans D, et al. Refinements in stress echocardiographic techniques improve inter-institutional agreement in interpretation of dobutamine stress echocardiograms. Eur Heart J 2002; 23:821–829.
22. Bjork Ingul C, Stoylen A, Slordahl SA, et al. Automated analysis of myocardial deformation at dobutamine stress echocardiography. An angiographic validation. J Am Coll Cardiol 2007; 49:1651–1659.
23. Franke A, Hoffmann R, Kuhl HP, et al. Non-contrast second harmonic imaging improves interobserver agreement and accuracy of dobutamine stress echocardiography in patients with impaired image quality. Heart 2000; 83:133–140.
24. Zamorano J, Sanchez V, Moreno R, et al. Contrast agents provide a faster learning curve in dipyridamole stress echocardiography. Int J Cardiovasc Imaging 2002; 18:415–419.
25. Varga A, Picano E, Dodi C, et al. Madness and method in stress echo reading. Eur Heart J 1999; 20:1271–1275.

26. Hoffmann R, Lethen H, Marwick T, et al. Standardized guidelines for the interpretation of dobutamine echocardiography reduce interinstitutional variance in interpretation. Am J Cardiol 1998; 82:1520–1524.
27. Imran MB, Palinkas A, Pasanisi EM, et al. Optimal reading criteria in stress echocardiography. Am J Cardiol 2002; 90:444–445.
28. Sicari R. Relevance of tissue Doppler in the quantification of stress echocardiography for the detection of myocardial ischemia in clinical practice. Cardiovasc Ultrasound 2005; 3:2.

5 | Stress Echocardiography: Protocols

Alja Vlahovic-Stipac, Biljana Putnikovic, and Aleksandar
N. Neskovic

*Department of Cardiology, Clinical-Hospital Center Zemun, Belgrade University
School of Medicine, Belgrade, Serbia*

For correct performance of stress echocardiography there are several procedures that have to be appreciated and applied generally to all stress modalities. These refer to patient preparation for the examination, technique of the specific test and the termination endpoints, either diagnostic or nondiagnostic.

First, patient should be placed in left lateral decubitus, allowing the best echocardiographic visualization, with electrocardiographic (ECG) leads placed on the chest wall for continuous ECG monitoring on the echo machine throughout the test. Also 12-lead ECG should be recorded before the test, at the end of each stage, and in recovery phase. For noninvasive blood pressure monitoring, the cuff should be placed on patient forearm and blood pressure measured at rest and at the end of every dose-step. In patients undergoing pharmacological stress echocardiography, intravenous access ideally should be enabled contralateral to the blood pressure cuff (1).

Nowadays, the majority of echo machines have predetermined protocols for the stress echocardiographic examination. These may be changed at physician's preference. Most frequently, so-called 4 × 4 protocol is used, consisting of four views, two apical (4- and 2-chamber views) and two parasternal (long- and short-axis views) recorded at four stages, usually at rest (baseline) and at the end of each stage. For pharmacological stress-echo, views are usually recorded twice during the test (at low and peak dose) and at recovery (post). Images can also be recorded in tissue velocity imaging mode (4 × 4 Q protocol) for off-line quantitative stress echocardiographic analysis (strain and strain-rate imaging). Feasibility of tissue velocity acquisition is the best in three apical views. Images are typically stored in "quad-screen" format. For the detection of inducible ischemia images stored at different stress stages are compared to each other in each echocardiographic view (1).

Although the images are being recorded intermittently, every effort should be made to perform echocardiographic evaluation continuously throughout the test, so the signs of ischemia could be noticed as early as they develop. This approach may prevent possible complications of prolonged ischemia and also enables risk stratification according to the stage at which ischemia has occurred (2).

Also, second harmonic imaging should always be applied for better visualization of endocardial borders. Better endocardial delineation of the left ventricle using contrast may further improve diagnostic performance, especially with less-experienced readers (3).

Digital image acquisition has to be used whenever possible, since it significantly improves image quality and allows side-by-side display for comparison of images recorded at different stages (4).

Importantly, the patient must be informed in details about the aim of the test, test protocol, and the symptoms that could probably be expected and are related to the specific stressor (i.e., flushing with dipyridamole, palpitations with dobutamine) and particularly the symptoms that may occur as a result of provoked ischemia (i.e., chest pain) (1).

Finally, when reporting the test results, not only information on left ventricular function and regional wall motion at different stages, but also the protocol used, the exercise time, maximal given dose of pharmacologic stressor, target and achieved heart rate, blood pressure response throughout the test, the reason for termination, symptoms, any complications, and ECG changes at peak versus baseline should be described (5).

Each stress echo test is performed until maximal workload is achieved, maximal dose of stressor is given, target heart rate is achieved (usually 85% of maximal heart rate predicted for age), or new or worsening wall motion abnormality develops. Such test is considered to be diagnostic for the detection of coronary artery disease. However, symptom intolerance (palpitations, headache, nausea, anxiety), severe hypertension (over 220/120 mm Hg) or persisting, serious supraventricular, or ventricular arrhythmias are considered as nondiagnostic endpoints requiring test termination. In these cases further diagnostic workup is usually required.

The development of severe hypotension ($\geq$20 mm Hg drop of blood pressure) during exercise stress echo is shown to be a marker of severe coronary artery disease (6). On the other hand, data on diagnostic significance of severe hypotension on dobutamine stress echocardiography (DSE) are equivocal. According to some reports, it may be the consequence of hyperdynamic left ventricle and intraventricular obstruction provoked by inotropic stimulation (7,8), not related to ischemia. Conversely, it can indicate poor ventricular functional reserve and predict cardiac death among patients with left ventricular dysfunction (9).

The occurrence of angina during stress echo is also a controversial issue in diagnostic terms. In patients without wall motion abnormality on DSE, it was shown to be associated with higher revascularization rate during long-term follow-up as compared to those without angina, but the incidence of cardiac death and nonfatal myocardial infarction was similar between the groups (10).

Another unresolved issue is the significance of ST-segment changes in patients without evidence of regional wall motion abnormality. It has been reported that these changes are not predictive of unfavorable long-term outcome (11).

I. PROTOCOLS

The protocols that are described in this chapter are related mostly to the detection and evaluation of coronary artery disease. Specific protocols applied for other conditions such as valvular heart diseases and dilated cardiomyopathy are presented in corresponding chapters.

Also, indications and contraindications for different stress echo tests are outlined in chapter 1, Table 4.

Intravenous route should be secured and resuscitation drugs and equipment must be ready for the use before starting any stress echo test. Continuous ECG monitoring and frequent blood pressure measurements are mandatory.

II. EXERCISE STRESS ECHOCARDIOGRAPHY

Among various imaging modalities, exercise stress echocardiography, as the most physiologic stressor, is the first line of choice, especially for the detection of coronary artery disease.

It may be performed using treadmill, and upright or supine bicycle.

Treadmill exercise stress test with standard Bruce protocol is frequently performed, but it has some disadvantages over the bicycle stress echo. For this test, images are acquired at baseline and just after the completion of exercise, with no information on left ventricular function in between. Also, the patient has to be moved from the treadmill to the imaging table immediately after the exercise, so that echo examination can be performed as soon as possible and the signs of ischemia (new or worsening asynergy) noticed before it resolves.

On the other hand, the potential problem with bicycle testing is that adequate test highly depends on patient cooperation and coordination, requiring constant cadence (55–60 rpm) with increasing workload (12,13). Protocol used for bicycle stress echocardiography is shown in Figure 1.

In upright bicycle, usually only apical and subcostal images may be acquired.

With the new ergometers allowing supine bicycle exercise with patient lying on the table that may be tilted leftwards, much better acquisition of echo images as well as continuous evaluation of different echo views throughout the

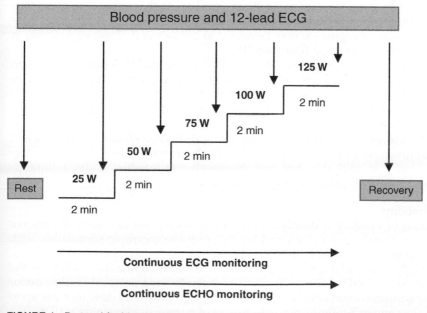

FIGURE 1 Protocol for bicycle stress echocardiography.

test are possible. According to recently published data, continuous echocardiographic examination with supine bicycle exercise significantly improves the sensitivity of the test for the detection of coronary artery disease (14).

A. Hemodynamic Changes

It is well known that exercise increases heart rate and blood pressure. However, the workload and maximum heart rate achieved tend to be higher with treadmill exercise, probably as a result of earlier leg fatigue development (15). On the other hand, ischemia usually occurs at lower workload with supine bicycle exercise, due to higher blood pressure and end-diastolic volume for the same level of stress at supine position.

B. Safety

Among various stress echo modalities exercise stress echocardiography is probably the safest, with overall complication rate of 0.09% (16) and extremely rare life-threatening complications occurring in only 1 in 6574 patients tested (17).

III. DOBUTAMINE STRESS ECHOCARDIOGRAPHY

A. Ischemia

In patients unable to exercise, pharmacological stress echo using adrenergic stimulation or vasodilators is a good alternative. Of adrenergic agents, dobutamine has been most frequently used. By stimulating mostly β_1-adrenergic receptors, it increases contractility and heart rate and may consequently induce ischemia in the presence of critical coronary artery stenosis.

The most widely used protocol for DSE includes the administration of dobutamine intravenously by infusion pump, starting with a dose of 5 μg/kg/min and increasing the dose up to 40 μg/kg/min, with incremental stages lasting 3 minutes each, as shown in Figure 2 (18). At the end of the highest dose of dobutamine, atropine i.v. may be added in boluses of 0.25 mg up to 2 mg, in order to achieve the target heart rate (19).

Recently, another protocol, the so-called accelerated DSE protocol has been introduced (20). This protocol proposes continuous dobutamine infusion of 50 μg/kg/min. It was shown to have good tolerability and safety, enabling the target heart rate to be reached in shorter time, without the need for atropine coadministration.

Whatever protocol is used, short-acting β-blocker should be on hand and may be given after the peak stress to slow the heart rate (5).

Also, it is advisable, but very frequently not feasible, to discontinue β-blocker therapy for at least 2 days before the test.

B. Viability

Detection of viability is mostly based on the assessment of contractile reserve in dysfunctional myocardium and for this purpose inotropic stimulation with dobutamine is most frequently used.

Both low- and high-dose protocols with dobutamine are useful for the evaluation of viability. Currently, most commonly used protocol implies dobutamine administration in initial dose of 2.5 μg/kg/min, with dose increase up to 20 μg/kg/min in 5-minute intervals. In case of no new or worsening wall motion abnormality, dose may be safely increased up to 40 μg/kg/min, so that ischemic and biphasic responses may be elicited (Fig. 3) (5).

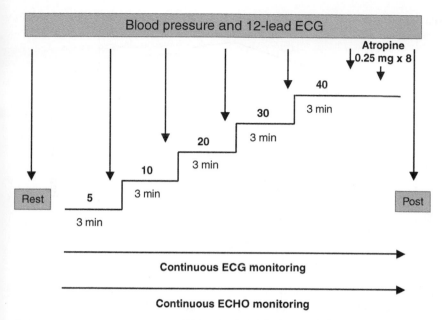

FIGURE 2 High-dose dobutamine protocol. The numbers refer to doses of dobutamine in μg/kg/min. As explained in the text, up to 2 mg of atropine is usually given if target heart rate is not achieved with highest dobutamine dose.

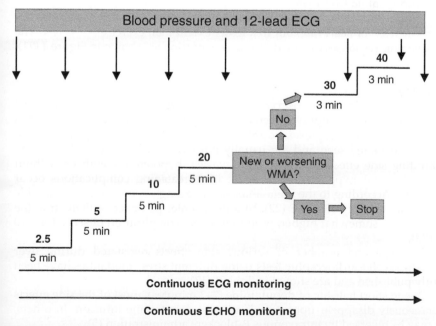

FIGURE 3 Dobutamine stress echo protocol for the assessment of viability. Doses are in μg/kg/min. *Abbreviation*: WMA, wall motion abnormality.

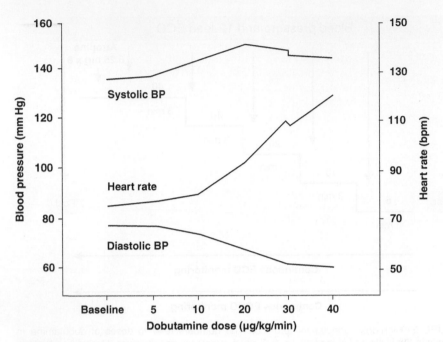

FIGURE 4 Changes in blood pressure and heart rate during high-dose dobutamine infusion. *Source*: From Ref. 21.

C. Hemodynamic Changes

Dobutamine infusion results in the increase of blood pressure and even more significant increase of heart rate, but to a lesser extent than exercise stress test. The hemodynamic responses during dobutamine infusion are shown in Figure 4 (21).

D. Safety

The majority of side effects observed during DSE are related to arrhythmogenic effect of dobutamine. Supraventricular and especially ventricular arrhythmias (frequent premature complexes, couplets, nonsustained ventricular tachycardia) are most frequently seen and are usually not ischemia induced. Other minor, but limiting side effects are: headache, nausea, hypotension with or without bradycardia, and hypertension. Serious, life-threatening complications occur quite rarely. According to the meta-analysis of 35 single centers one serious side effect occurs in every 335 DSE (22). In a multicenter prospective EDIC trial the incidence was somewhat higher, with one severe complication observed in 210 DSE (23).

The type and number of serious side effects registered during over 85,000 stress echocardiographic tests using different stress modalities have been recently published and are shown in Table 1 (17).

Due to short half-life of dobutamine (2–3 minutes), most of the side effects spontaneously disappear upon termination of dobutamine infusion. In others, they may be reversed by intravenous β-blockers administration (5).

TABLE 1 Serious Side Effects of Different Stress Echo Tests Registered During Over 85,000 Stress Echocardiographic Tests

Complication	Dobutamine	Dipyridamole	Exercise
Acute MI	11	5	1
Sustained VT	27	1	2
Ventricular fibrillation	11	2	0
Cardiac rupture	5	0	1
Asystole	2	4	0
TIA/stroke	3	3	0
Hypotension/shock	2	4	0
Third degree AV block	2	0	0

Abbreviations: AV, atrioventricular; MI, myocardial infarction; TIA, transitory ischemic attack; VT, ventricular tachycardia.
Source: From Ref. 17.

IV. DIPYRIDAMOLE STRESS ECHOCARDIOGRAPHY

In patients with contraindications to dobutamine stress echo test (complex atrial and ventricular arrhythmias, moderate-to-severe hypertension), dipyridamole with its hyperemic and proischemic effects is a useful stress modality for the diagnosis of coronary artery disease or for the detection of viable myocardium.

Before the test patient should be advised not to take any caffeine-containing foods at least 12 hours before the test. Also, medications containing theophylline (such as aminophylline) should be withdrawn for at least 24 hours (24). These drugs block adenosine receptors which are the main site of action of dipyridamole as well as adenosine.

As opposed to other pharmacological stressors, dipyridamole is usually infused with hand-held syringe.

A. Ischemia

For detection of ischemia, dipyridamole is administered in dose of 0.84 mg/kg over 10 minutes, alone or with 1-mg atropine coadministration (25,26). Also, a so-called "fast protocol," with 6-minute infusion of same dipyridamole dose may be used (Fig. 5).

Sometimes, dipyridamole may be combined with exercise or dobutamine to increase the test sensitivity for the detection of milder forms of coronary artery disease (27,28). However, these tests are time-consuming, patient demanding, may be misleading in terms of detection of some clinically insignificant stenosis, and are therefore not recommended for routine practice.

Aminophylline should routinely be given to all patients at the end of the test, even if it is negative. However, since the half-life of dipyridamole is 6 hours, the symptoms may reoccur later.

B. Viability

The assessment of viability using dipyridamole is based on its ability to produce hyperemia, especially when given in very low doses. The dose of 0.28 mg/kg predominantly increases the coronary flow, with virtually no ischemic effect (29).

The protocol of low-dose dipyridamole is shown in Figure 5.

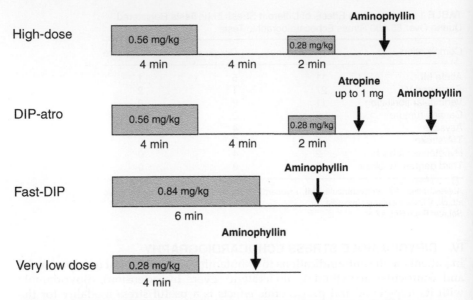

FIGURE 5 Different protocols for dipyridamole stress echocardiography test. The upper three protocols are used for induction of ischemia. Protocol presented at the bottom is usually applied for identification of viable myocardium. *Abbreviations*: Atro, atropine; DIP, dipyridamole. *Source*: From Ref. 24.

C. Hemodynamic Effects

Dipyridamole usually slightly increases heart rate and induces mild-to-moderate decrease of blood pressure.

D. Safety

Safety of dipyridamole stress echo test has been well documented. Minor but limiting side effects, manifested as hypotension and/or bradycardia, headache, dizziness, or nausea occur in 5% of patients, with about 60% of patients experiencing effects resulting from dipyridamole-induced vasodilatation, such as flushing and headache (24). According to the results of EPIC study, life-threatening complications occurred in 1 out of 1500 tests, with 1 fatal outcome in every 10,000 studies (30).

The majority of these side effects may be reversed by aminophylline. Rarely, ischemia may persist despite the aminophylline administration and in such cases nitrates should be given (31). The same treatment is recommended in case of aminophylline-induced coronary vasospasm (32).

Note: *The following four stress echo modalities have not been evaluated broadly and some of them (like transesophageal pacing) have been abandoned. Still, according to the data from the literature each of these tests can be applied for diagnostic evaluation of coronary artery disease, especially in certain subset of patients or for specific forms of coronary artery disease. Therefore, they are also described in this chapter. However, it should be emphasized that these modalities are rarely used and are of limited value in routine clinical practice.*

V. ADENOSINE STRESS ECHOCARDIOGRAPHY

Like dipyridamole, adenosine is a vasodilator, expressing its effect by direct stimulation of A_2 receptors in coronary arteries. It has a half-life of only few seconds, which is much shorter than that of dipyridamole and therefore aminophylline administration is rarely required (33).

A. Ischemia

This test is mostly used for the detection of ischemia, although there are some data on its usefulness for viability assessment (34). The protocol for adenosine stress echo is shown in Figure 6.

B. Hemodynamic Effects

Like dipyridamole, adenosine administration is associated with slight increase in heart rate and usually mild decrease in systemic arterial pressure (35).

C. Safety

Adenosine stress echocardiography is associated with quite frequent minor, but limiting side effects, with the incidence of up to 25% (36,37). Of those, high-degree atrioventricular block, hypotension, intolerable chest pain, flushing, and headaches are most commonly seen. Usually, they disappear with the discontinuation of adenosine infusion.

Although minor adverse reactions occur more frequently and are less well tolerated than with other pharmacological stressors, life-threatening side effects are rare, observed in less than 0.01% of examinations (37).

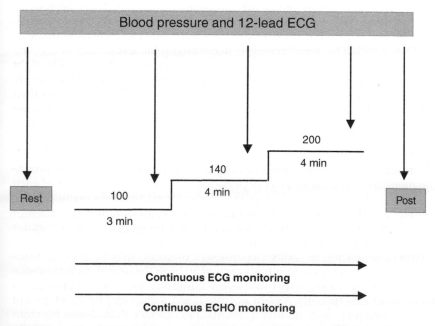

FIGURE 6 Standard protocol for adenosine stress echocardiographic test. Doses are in µg/kg/min.

VI. PACING STRESS ECHOCARDIOGRAPHY

For the assessment of coronary artery disease either transesophageal atrial pacing or noninvasive pacing in patients with permanent pacemaker may be used. In case of transesophageal pacing left atrium is a paced chamber and in patients with permanent pacemaker either right atrium or right ventricle may be stimulated (38).

Pacing stress echocardiography is considered by some as an efficient, inexpensive, and faster alternative to the pharmacologic stressors (39,40), with similar diagnostic accuracy to other stress modalities (41).

A. Transesophageal Atrial Pacing

The patient preparation for this type of stress echocardiography is quite different than for other previously described tests. First, patient should be fasting for 3 to 4 hours before the test. Local oropharyngeal or nasopharyngeal anesthesia is almost always applied. In anxious patient intravenous midazolam may be given for sedation (42).

The cardiac pacing and recording catheter (inserted through a 10F sheath) are advanced through oropharynx or nasopharynx by having the patient swallow while in the left lateral decubitus position. The catheter is positioned to about 40 ± 4 cm, depending on the site of insertion.

Appropriate capture of the atrial rhythm is depicted by maximal amplitude of the esophageal P wave on the ECG, at the lowest current that provides stable atrial capture ($\sim$10 mA) (Fig. 7) (42).

B. Noninvasive Pacing in Patients with Permanent Pacemaker

In patients with permanent ventricular pacemaker, ECG is usually useless for noninvasive diagnostic evaluation of ischemic heart disease. In these patients, ischemia may be induced by programming the pacemaker to increasing frequencies and it is detected by simultaneous echocardiographic assessment of regional left ventricular function. However, since septal motion is usually altered by right ventricular pacing, the assessment of inducible ischemia should predominantly be based on the analysis of wall thickening, which is much less affected then wall motion (43). With right atrial pacing there are no special interpretation difficulties.

C. Protocols

Blood pressure should be recorded in every 2 minutes and heart rate is continuously monitored. A 12-lead ECG is performed at baseline, at the end of each stage or at peak heart rate, and immediately after the pacing. Echocardiographic images are recorded at rest, at the end of each stage, and upon termination of pacing, with the last recording before recovery phase being made after 3 minutes of pacing at the highest achieved heart rate.

With either pacing modality two different protocols may be applied. Standard protocol refers to a starting frequency of 10 bpm (beats per minute) above basal value and increasing heart rate every 2 minutes by 10 to 20 bpm up to the target heart rate (usually, 85% of age predicted maximum) or development of new or worsening wall motion abnormalities, greater than 2-mm horizontal or downsloping ST-segment depression, or intolerable symptoms, especially angina (5,38,42). In accelerated protocol, the test usually begins with a heart rate

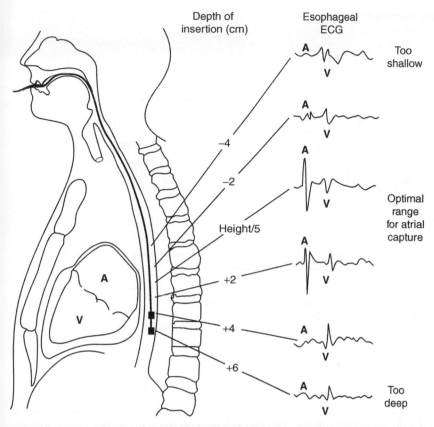

FIGURE 7 Schematic presentation, showing appropriate position of pacing wire with corresponding electrocardiographic tracing of transesophageal atrial pacing. Inadequate atrial recordings requiring repositioning of cardiac pacing and recording catheter are also shown. *Source*: From Ref. 42.

of 120/bpm and it is increased in every 20 to 30 seconds up to target heart rate (Fig. 8) (42).

D. Hemodynamic Effects

An increase in heart rate induced by atrial pacing produces an increase in myocardial oxygen demand with mild increase or no change in blood pressure (44).

E. Safety

Due to the ability to instantly lower heart rate and terminate test, this is a very safe stress modality. In a large series of over 1700 tests with transesophageal atrial pacing, no life-threatening complication was observed (45). Minor side effects, mostly self-limiting supraventricular arrhythmias, were observed in only 1.6% of patients.

Example: Baseline HR 90/min

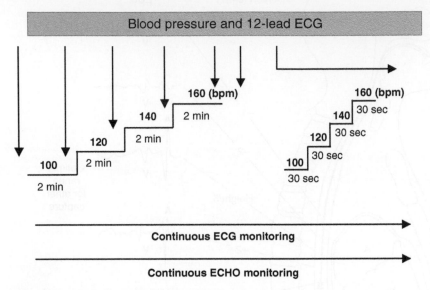

FIGURE 8   Standard and accelerated protocols for pacing stress echocardiography.

VII.   ERGONOVINE STRESS ECHOCARDIOGRAPHY

Although typically detected by provocative procedures during coronary angiography, coronary vasospasm may also be reliably diagnosed using noninvasive bedside ergonovine stress echocardiography (46), even in patients with almost normal angiographic findings. The test is based on the echocardiographic assessment of regional left ventricular function and detection of new wall motion abnormalities after administration of ergonovine. The results obtained with this test have significant prognostic implications in patients without fixed coronary stenoses (47).

A.   Protocol

β-Blockers, calcium channel blocker, and long-acting nitrates should be discontinued for at least five half-lives before the test (46).

Standard protocol for ergonovine stress echocardiography implies the administration of ergonovine bolus i.v. in dose of 50 μg initially, and subsequently 50 μg boluses at 5-minute intervals, up to the maximum dose of 350 μg. The development of new wall motion abnormality or ST-segment elevation/depression suggests the occurrence of coronary vasospasm (Fig. 9). The occurrence of significant arrhythmias, hyper/hypotension may also require termination of the test.

In modified protocol, after initial bolus of 50 μg, test is proceeded with further boluses of 100 μg up to 350 μg.

If abnormal response is detected, intravenous bolus injection of nitroglycerine (0.25 mg) should immediately be administered. Due to half-life of ergonovine

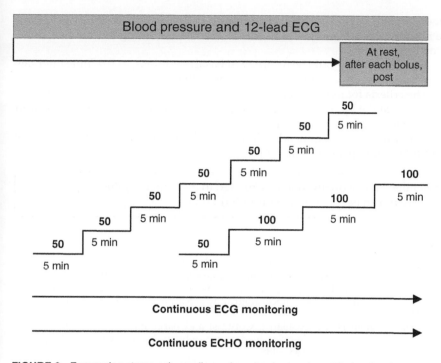

FIGURE 9 Ergonovine stress echocardiography: standard and modified protocols.

of 30 to 116 minutes (48), sublingual 10 mg of nifedipine may also be given to prevent possible delayed effect of ergonovine.

B. Safety

Two major disadvantages of noninvasive versus invasive spasm-provocation tests are that intracoronary nitroglycerine cannot be given if needed and that the placement of temporary pacemaker is much less feasible.

In a large series of over 1300 patients, no life-threatening complications were observed (49). Also, the incidence of transient and reversible significant arrhythmias and atrioventricular block was low, occurring in about 2% of tests. In another study, ischemia independent events such as hyper/hypotension, nausea, and vomiting developed in 3% of patients studied (50).

VIII. HYPERVENTILATION TEST

As an alternative to ergonovine stress echocardiography, hyperventilation test alone or in combination with exercise and cold-pressor test may also be used for detection of coronary spasm (51–53).

A. Protocol

For provocation of vasospasm, patient is advised to breath deeply with frequency of 25/min to 30/min for 5 minutes. In susceptible patients, coronary spasm will usually develop 1 to 5 minutes after cessation of hyperventilation. In combined hyperventilation and cold-pressor test, immediately after hyperventilation period, cold-pressor stress may be administered by submerging the patient's right hand in ice water for 2 minutes (52). Another possibility is to combine mild hyperventilation with treadmill exercise according to modified Bruce protocol (53).

A 12-lead ECG should be recorded at basal conditions, at 1-minute intervals during the stress test, and for 15 minutes thereafter.

The criteria for terminating the stress test are an ST-segment shift of greater than 0.1 mV at the J-point, occurrence of chest pain, or development of new wall motion abnormality.

The test is not recommended in physically deconditioned patients and is contraindicated in patients with epilepsy.

> **DVD note:** The following loops are related to the content of this chapter: 1–33. These loops can be found in the provided DVD.

REFERENCES

1. Picano E. Stress echocardiography: Instruction for use. In: Picano E, ed. Stress Echocardiography. Heidelberg, Berlin: Springer-Verlag, 2003:91–101.
2. Das M, Pellikka P, Mahoney D, et al. Assessment of cardiac risk before nonvascular surgery: Dobutamine stress echocardiography in 530 patients. J Am Coll Cardiol 2000; 35:1647–1653.
3. Vlassak I, Rubin D, Odabashian J. Contrast and harmonic imaging improves the accuracy and efficiency of novice readers for dobutamine stress echocardiography. Echocardiography 2002; 19:483–488.
4. Feigenbaum H. Digital recording, display, and storage of echocardiograms. J Am Soc Echocardiogr 1988; 1:378–383.
5. Pellikka PA, Nagueh SH, Elhendy AA, et al. American Society of Echocardiography recommendations for performance, interpretation, and application of stress echocardiography. J Am Soc Echocardiogr 2008; 21:337–341.
6. Dubach P, Froelicher VF, Klein J, et al. Exercise-induced hypotension in a male population. Criteria, causes, and prognosis. Circulation 1988; 78(6):1380–1387.
7. Siddiqui TS, Dawn B, Stoddard MF. Hypotension during dobutamine stress transesophageal echocardiography: Relationship with provoked left ventricular obstruction. J Am Soc Echocardiogr 2006; 19:1144–1149.
8. Rallidis LS, Moyssakis IE, Nihoyannopoulos P. Hypotensive response during dobutamine stress echocardiography in coronary patients: A common event of well-functioning left ventricle. Clin Cardiol 1998; 21:747–752.
9. Wang CH, Cherng WJ, Hung MJ. Dobutamine-induced hypotension is an independent predictor for mortality in patients with left ventricular dysfunction following myocardial infarction. Int J Cardiol 1999; 68(3):297–302.
10. Elhendy A, Biagini E, Schinkel AF, et al. Clinical and prognostic implications of angina pectoris developing during dobutamine stress echocardiography in the absence of inducible wall motion abnormalities. Am J Cardiol 2005; 96:788–793.
11. Dhond MR, Nguyen T, Whitley TB, et al. Prognostic value of 12-lead electrocardiogram during dobutamine stress echocardiography. Echocardiography 2000; 17:429–432.
12. Roger V, Pellikka P, Oh J, et al. Stress echocardiography, Part I: Exercise echocardiography; techniques, implementation, clinical applications, and correlations. Mayo Clin Proc 1995; 70:5–15.
13. Picano E. Exercise echocardiography. In: Picano E, ed. Stress Echocardiography. Heidelberg, Berlin: Springer-Verlag, 2003:103–114.
14. Park TH, Tayan N, Takeda K, et al. Improved diagnostic accuracy and physiologic assessment of coronary artery disease with the incorporation of intermediate stages of exercise. J Am Coll Cardiol 2007; 50:1857–1863.

15. Thadani U, West RO, Mathew TM, et al. Hemodynamics at rest and during supine and sitting bicycle exercise in patients with coronary artery disease. Am J Cardiol 1977; 39:776–783.
16. Kane GC, Hepinstall MJ, Kidd GM, et al. Safety of stress echocardiography supervised by registered nurses: Results of a 2-year audit of 15404 patients. J Am Soc Echocardiogr 2008; 21:337–341.
17. Varga A, Garcia MR, Picano E. Safety of stress echocardiography from the international stress echo complication registry. Am J Cardiol 2006; 98:541–543.
18. Sawada S, Segar D, Ryan T, et al. Echocardiographic detection of coronary artery disease during dobutamine infusion. Circulation 1991; 83:1605–1614.
19. Ling L, Pellikka P, Mahoney D, et al. Atropine augmentation in dobutamine stress echocardiography: Role and incremental value in a clinical practice setting. J Am Coll Cardiol 1996; 28:551–557.
20. Minardi G, Manzara C, Pulignano G, et al. Feasibility, safety and tolerability of accelerated dobutamine stress echocardiography. Cardiovasc Ultrasound 2007; 5:40–46.
21. Hays JT, Mahmarian JJ, Cochran AJ, et al. Dobutamine thallium-201 tomography for evaluating patients with suspected coronary artery disease unable to undergo exercise or vasodilator pharmacologic stress testing. J Am Coll Cardiol 1993; 21:1583–1590.
22. Mathias W Jr, Arruda A, Santos F, et al. Safety of dobutamine–atropine stress echocardiography: A prospective experience of 4033 consecutive studies. J Am Soc Echocardiogr 1999; 12:785–791.
23. Picano E, Mathias W Jr, Pingitore A, et al. On behalf of the Echo-Dobutamine International Cooperative Study Group. Safety and tolerability of dobutamine–atropine stress echocardiography: A prospective multicentre study. Lancet 1994; 29:1190–1192.
24. Picano E. Dipyridamole stress echocardiography. In: Picano E, ed. Stress Echocardiography. Heidelberg, Berlin: Springer-Verlag, 2003:133–153.
25. Picano E, Lattanzi F, Masini M, et al. High dose dipyridamole echocardiography test in effort angina pectoris. Am J Cardiol 1986; 8:848–854.
26. Picano E, Pingatore A, Conti U, et al. Enhanced sensitivity for detection of coronary artery disease by addition of atropine to dipyridamole echocardiography. Eur Heart J 1993; 14:1216–1222.
27. Picano E, Lattanzi F, Masini M, et al. Usefulness of the dipyridamole-exercise echocardiography test for diagnosis of coronary artery disease. Am J Cardiol 1986; 62:67–70.
28. Ostojic M, Picano B, Beleslin B, et al. Dipyridamole-dobutamine echocardiography: A novel test for the detection of milder forms of coronary artery disease. J Am Coll Cardiol 1994; 23:1115–1122.
29. Picano E. Dipyridamole-echocardiography test: Historical background and physiologic basis. Eur Heart J 1989; 10:365–376.
30. Picano E, Marini C, Pirelli S, et al. Safety of intravenous high-dose dipyridamole echocardiography. The Echo-Persantine International Cooperative Study Group. Am J Cardiol 1992; 70:252–258.
31. Picano E, Lattanzi F, Distante A, et al. Role of myocardial oxygen consumption in dipyridamole-induced ischemia. Am Heart J 1989; 118:314–319.
32. Picano E, Lattanzi F, Masini M, et al. Aminophylline termination of dipyridamole stress as a trigger of coronary vasospasm in variant angina. Am J Cardiol 1988; 62:694–697.
33. Cerqueira MD, Verani MS, Schwaiger M, et al. Safety profile of adenosine stress perfusion imaging: Results from adenosan multicenter trial registry. J Am Coll Cardiol 1994; 23:384–389.
34. Case RA, Buckmire R, McLaughlin DP, et al. Physiological assessment of coronary artery disease and myocardial viability in ischemic syndromes using adenosine echocardiography. Echocardiography 1994; 11:133–143.
35. Iskandrian AS, Verani MS, Heo J. Pharmacological stress testing: Mechanism of action, hemodynamic responses and results in detection of coronary artery disease. J Nucl Cardiol 1994; 1:94–111.
36. Marwick T, Willemart B, D'Hondt AM, et al. Selection of optimal nonexercise stress for the evaluation of ischemic regional myocardial dysfunction and malperfusion.

Comparison of dobutamine and adenosine using echocardiography and ^{99m}Tc-MIBI single photon emission computed tomography. Circulation 1993; 87:345–354.

37. Djordjevic-Dikic A, Ostojic MC, Beleslin BD, et al. High-dose adenosine stress echocardiography for noninvasive detection of coronary artery disease. J Am Coll Cardiol 1996; 28:1689–1695.

38. Picano E. Pacing stress echocardiography. In: Picano E, ed. Stress Echocardiography. Heidelberg, Berlin: Springer-Verlag, 2003:165–171.

39. Chapman PD, Doyle TP, Troup PJ, et al. Stress echocardiography with trans-esophageal atrial pacing: Preliminary report of a new method for detection of ischemic wall motion abnormalities. Circulation 1984; 70:445–455.

40. Atar S, Nagai T, Cercek B, et al. Pacing stress echocardiography: An alternative to pharmacologic stress testing. J Am Coll Cardiol 2000; 36:1935–1941.

41. Schroder K, Voller H, Dingerkus H, et al. Comparison of the diagnostic potential of four echocardiographic stress tests shortly after acute myocardial infarction: Submaximal exercise, transesophageal atrial pacing, dipyridamole, and dobutamine-atropine. Am J Cardiol 1996; 77:909–914.

42. Modi SA, Siegel RJ, Birnbaum Y, et al. Systematic overview and clinical applications of pacing atrial stress echocardiography. Am J Cardiol 2006; 98:549–556.

43. Gomes JA, Damato AN, Akhtar M, et al. Ventricular septal motion and left ventricular dimensions during abnormal ventricular activation. Am J Cardiol 1977; 39:641–650.

44. O'Brien KP, Higgs LM, Glancy DL, et al. Hemodynamic accompaniments of angina: A comparison during angina induced by exercise and by atrial pacing. Circulation 1969; 39:735–743.

45. Anselmi M, Golia G, Rossi A, et al. Feasibility and safety of transesophageal atrial pacing stress echocardiography in patients with known or suspected coronary artery disease. Am J Cardiol 2003; 92:1384–1388.

46. Song JK, Lee SJK, Kang DH, et al. Ergonovine echocardiography as a screening test for diagnosis of vasospastic angina before coronary angiography. J Am Coll Cardiol 1996; 27:1156–1161.

47. Song JK, Park SW, Kang DH, et al. Prognostic implication of ergonovine echocardiography in patients with near normal coronary angiogram or negative stress test for significant fixed stenosis. J Am Soc Echocardiogr 2002; 15:1346–1352.

48. Mantyla R, Kanto J. Clinical pharmacokinetic of methylergometrine (methylergonovine). Int J Clin Pharmacol Biopharm 1981; 19:386–391.

49. Song JK, Park SW, Kang DH, et al. Safety and clinical impact of ergonovine stress echocardiography for diagnosis of coronary vasospasm. J Am Coll Cardiol 2000; 35:1850–1856.

50. Pálinkás A, Picano E, Rodriguez O, et al. Safety of ergot stress echocardiography for non-invasive detection of coronary vasospasm. Coron Artery Dis 2001; 12:649–654.

51. Picano E. Hyperventilation test. In: Picano E, ed. Stress Echocardiography. Heidelberg, Berlin: Springer-Verlag, 2003:183–187.

52. Hirano Y, Ozasa Y, Yamamoto T, et al. Hyperventilation and cold-pressor stress echocardiography for noninvasive diagnosis of coronary artery spasm. J Am Soc Echo 2001; 14:626–633.

53. Sueda S, Fukuda H, Watanabe K, et al. Usefulness of accelerated exercise following mild hyperventilation for the induction of coronary artery spasm: Comparison with an acetylcholine test. Chest 2001; 119:155–162.

Detection of Myocardial Ischemia

Manish Bansal and Thomas H. Marwick

University of Queensland, Brisbane, Australia

Since its introduction about 30 years ago, stress echocardiography has evolved into an established clinical tool for the diagnostic and prognostic assessment of patients with suspected or known coronary artery disease. Although an extensive evidence base supports its use in a variety of clinical settings, detection of coronary artery disease remains the primary indication for its performance.

For the diagnosis of coronary artery disease, stress echocardiography can be performed in conjunction with a number of different stressors. The hemodynamic effects of the various stressors, their side effects, and the protocols for their use have already been discussed in previous chapters. This chapter will focus on the use of different modes of stress echocardiography for detection of myocardial ischemia and relative merits of the different techniques for this purpose.

I. PATHOPHYSIOLOGY

Stress echocardiography is based on the induction of regional wall motion abnormalities by provoking regional mismatch between myocardial blood supply and myocardial oxygen demand in the presence of obstructive coronary artery disease. When subjected to increased workload induced by exercise or inotropic stress, the left ventricle normally responds by an increase in the endocardial excursion and myocardial thickening with consequent increase in ejection fraction and a reduction in end-systolic cavity size. However, when the blood supply to one or more myocardial segments is compromised, the affected segments fail to improve contractile function. Although failure to augment as much as adjacent segments has been used in the past as a marker of ischemia, this finding alone is sensitive but not specific, and our practice is to identify these as abnormal if there is also delayed contraction. Delayed (but still adequate) thickening is the earliest finding with ischemia, followed by reduced thickening, and finally no thickening at all. These abnormalities of regional wall motion are the echocardiographic hallmarks of ischemia and their recognition forms the basis for the performance of stress echocardiography. More severe ischemia is characterized by enlargement of LV cavity size and reduction in ejection fraction. These ischemic changes are usually short lasting and disappear promptly with cessation of stress. However, more severe ischemia may lead to myocardial stunning in which case the changes may last for as long as 30 minutes or even longer following stress.

II. INTERPRETATION OF STRESS ECHOCARDIOGRAPHY

Despite the development of techniques for quantitation of stress echocardiography, the standard approach to the interpretation of stress echocardiogram continues to be based on qualitative assessment of regional wall motion before, during, and following stress. The subjectivity of this process is responsible for several of the limitations of stress echocardiography. The most important of these is the need for extensive expertise in both the performance and interpretation of stress echocardiography to ensure accurate results (1). Even skilled echocardiographers need to undergo additional training in stress echocardiography in order to provide accurate reading of stress echocardiograms, and this requirement is of course greater in the case of novice readers. Although the exact details and duration of the requisite training are undefined (and in any case will vary with individual circumstance), the available evidence suggests that experience with at least 100 studies is necessary in order to raise the accuracy of the novice readers to expert level (2), and regular exposure is then required to maintain and further enhance this skill.

The second problem that arises from the subjective nature of stress echocardiography interpretation relates to its reproducibility. Although good reproducibility is often reported among readers from the same centers, even in the hands of experienced readers, interinstitutional agreement remains suboptimal (3). Concordance can be enhanced by improved image quality, side-by-side display, and standard reading criteria (4,5). A systematic step-by-step approach to the interpretation of stress echocardiography has therefore been recommended with the view to reduce subjectivity and to improve the reproducibility of the test.

The reading of a stress echocardiogram should begin with an evaluation of the resting images including M-mode and color Doppler. Resting regional wall motion should be scored using the 16-segment model recommended by the American Society of the Echocardiography or the 17-segment model proposed by the American Heart Association. Our practice remains to use the former because the true apex is often excluded from the "apical" images. Accurate identification of regional wall motion at rest is critical in determining the stress response and therefore adequate attention and time should be spent in evaluation of the resting function. Of particular significance is the differentiation between akinesis and hypokinesis at rest. Segments that are truly akinetic at rest cannot be identified as ischemic unless a protocol is used that permits detection of augmentation at low-level stress (dobutamine, dipyridamole, or cycle ergometry). In the absence of this, any deterioration in function with stress (e.g., the development of dyskinesis) is usually a result of altered loading conditions rather than a result of induction of ischemia (6). Hypokinetic segments may remain unchanged, improve, or deteriorate in function following stress. Improvement in contractile function with stress suggests the segment to be normal whereas worsening with stress (whether at low or high threshold) is a marker of ischemia. The differentiation between akinetic and hypokinetic segments at rest is easier if there is increased echodensity or thinning of the wall as these are highly suggestive of scarring and thus akinesis. In the absence of these, a thickening of <10% during systole is suggestive of akinesia. An endocardial excursion of <2 mm has also been proposed as a marker of akinesia but is less reliable than wall thickening as it may result from tethering by adjacent segments. Following a meticulous assessment of the regional systolic function, global LV systolic function should be assessed either by calculation of wall motion score index or measurement of ejection fraction.

The evaluation of the stress images should start with a technical assessment of the digital images, to ensure adequate image quality, appropriate triggering, and comparability of views at each stage. An assessment of LV size and shape may yield clues about abnormal global stress responses, as may be seen in valvular heart disease, cardiomyopathies, or extensive ischemia (Fig. 1). This

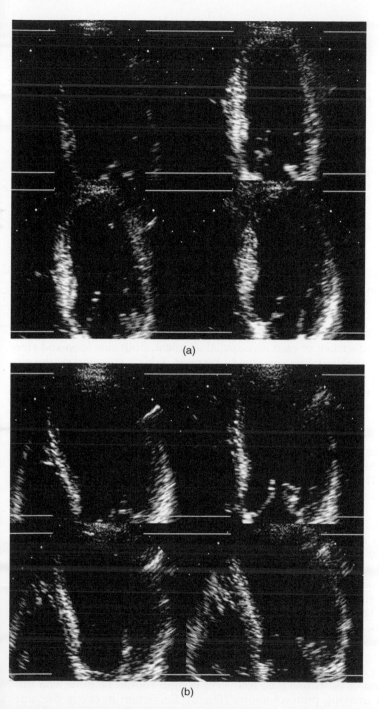

(a)

(b)

FIGURE 1 Response of global LV function to exercise. The normal response (**A**) involves reduction of LV volumes and an increment of EF. Failure to reduce LV volumes or increment EF (**B**) denotes loss of contractile reserve (loops 32 and 33).

TABLE 1   Interpretation of Exercise and Pharmacologic Stress Echocardiography

Nature of tissue	Resting function	Low dose	Peak/poststress function
Normal	Normal	Normal	Hyperkinetic
Ischemic	Normal	Normal (may worsen with severe CAD)	Worse than rest
			Worse than adjacent segments Tardokinesis (delayed contraction)
Viable, ischemic	Rest WMA	Improvement at low dose	Reduction (compared with low dose)
Viable, nonischemic	Rest WMA	Improvement at low dose	Sustained improvement
Infarction	Rest WMA	No change	No change

Abbreviations: CAD, coronary artery disease; WMA, wall motion abnormalities (severe hypokinesis, akinesis, and dyskinesis).

finding is more common with exercise echocardiography and is often masked by the reduction in afterload with dobutamine (7). Regional LV shape change is another useful clue to the presence of ischemia and should alert the interpreter to the presence of coronary disease.

After global evaluation of poststress images, careful side-by-side analysis should be undertaken of each myocardial segment. Both cine loop and stop frame review of the digital images should be used. Table 1 summarizes the criteria for the interpretation of the regional stress response. All segments should be carefully analyzed for the presence of reduced wall thickening or delayed contraction compared to rest. Emphasis should be placed on assessment of wall thickening rather than wall motion or endocardial excursion as these may result from tethering or translational movement of the heart. Stepping through the individual frames to assess the extent and speed of thickening in the first half of systole is important, as this phase is relatively independent of translational motion and tethering. The evaluation of short-axis images is often helpful, as it may overcome problems related to off-axis imaging and also when apical window is not adequate.

While analyzing individual segments, the vascular distribution of the different coronary arteries should be kept in consideration as the ischemic abnormalities usually follow these vascular territories (Fig. 2). Atypical patterns (e.g., involving mid-wall ischemia with apical preservation) may be seen following revascularization. Beware of apparent involvement of single segments, especially at peak stress, and especially if unverified from other views. Particular care should be taken during the evaluation of basal inferoseptal and lateral walls as false-positive results are common in the former and false negatives in the latter (8). Abnormalities (or their absence) in these regions should be corroborated with the findings in the other segments supplied by the same vascular territory before reaching any conclusion (Table 2).

Evaluation of poststress (i.e., recovery) images should be done as a routine whenever imaging protocol allows (Fig. 3). Reduction in cavity size during stress (especially with dobutamine) may mask development of ischemia and result in a false-negative study unless poststress images (or reversal of

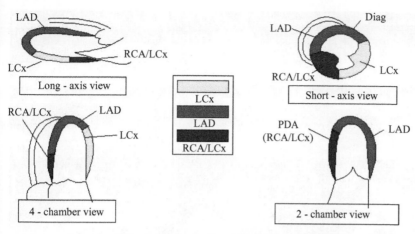

1 = normal; 2 = hypokinetic; 3 = akinetic; 4 = dyskinetic

FIGURE 2 Distribution of coronary perfusion territories, according to 16-segment LV model.

dobutamine-induced tachycardia with β-blockers) allow enlargement of the cavity, thus inducing ischemia (or making it more apparent). Some exercise stress echo protocols do not allow acquisition of recovery images—in this case, extra images might be saved on videotape. Review of videotaped stress images has been shown to increase the accuracy of stress echo interpretation (9). Unfortunately, the lack of random access to studies can make this time-consuming; most of the benefit of this step is derived from its use in patients with poor-quality images or when there is uncertainty regarding the final diagnosis. Unlike digital cine loops that are limited by the ability to store representative cardiac cycles in only the standard views, continuous videotape recording is often helpful in allowing assessment in intermediate views.

Finally, and depending on the clinical scenario, data additional to wall motion may be of value. This may include the evaluation of mitral regurgitation or aortic stenosis, or the measurement of LV filling pressures using the ratio of annular and transmitral Doppler velocities. With the recognition that dyspnea may be an angina-equivalent, this is an important confirmatory step for diastolic heart failure (Fig. 4).

TABLE 2 Causes of False-Negative and False-Positive Stress Echocardiograms

False negatives	False positives
Inadequate stress	Localized basal inferior wall abnormalities
Antianginal treatment (especially β-blocker)	Overinterpretation (interpreter bias)
Mild stenosis	Hypertensive response to stress
Left circumflex disease	Abnormal septal motion (LBBB, post-CABG)
Delayed images poststress	Cardiomyopathies
Poor image quality	

Abbreviations: CABG, coronary artery bypass grafting; LBBB, left bundle branch block.

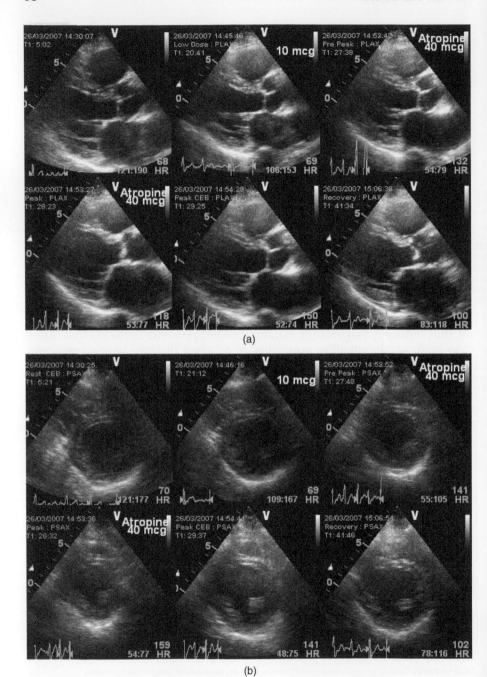

(a)

(b)

FIGURE 3 Multivessel disease. Each level of stress (rest, low dose, prepeak, two peak, and recovery) is viewed in the parasternal long axis (**A**), short axis (**B**), and apical 4 (**C**), 2 (**D**), and long axis (**E**). The LV enlarges with stress. Hypokinesis in the LAD territory (septum, anteroseptum, and anterior) develops at prepeak, while lateral changes are identified in recovery (loops 34–38).

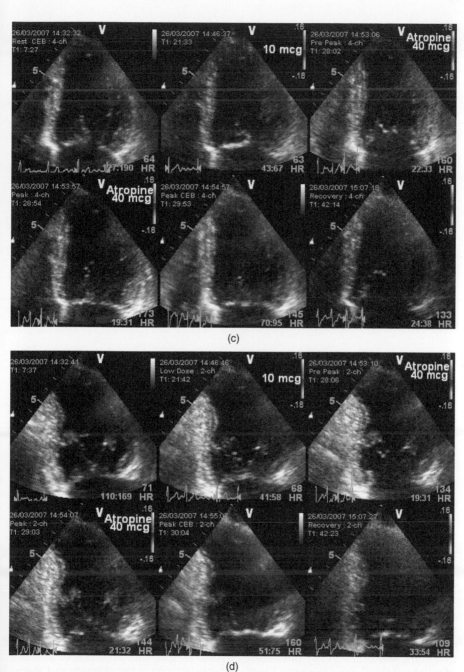

(c)

(d)

FIGURE 3 (*Continued*)

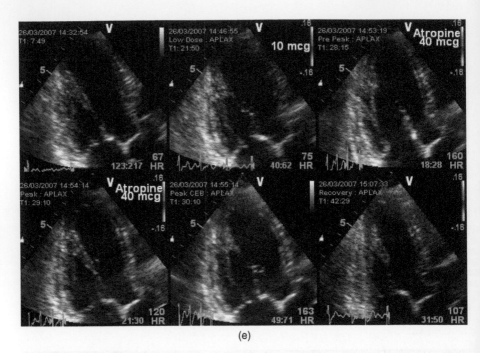

(e)

FIGURE 3   (*Continued*)

The final stress echocardiography report should include information about the presence or absence of ischemia, site and extent of ischemia, and the threshold of ischemia (in case of pharmacological stressors) in addition to the LV function and hemodynamic data. Other abnormalities detected at rest or during stress should also be mentioned in the final report.

III.   ACCURACY OF STRESS ECHOCARDIOGRAPHY

A.   Factors Influencing the Accuracy of Stress Echocardiography

Lesion Severity

The accuracy of functional testing for detection of myocardial ischemia is traditionally assessed by comparison with angiographic coronary artery disease (with "significant" stenoses being defined as >50–70% in diameter). The use of different cutoffs for angiographic severity of the disease influences the accuracy of functional testing, with a higher sensitivity and lower specificity for detection of disease when a higher cutoff is used for defining disease. Several factors in addition to the stenosis severity (including stenosis length, site, presence, or absence of collateral flow) determine the functional significance of the stenosis and therefore the correlation between anatomic and a physiologic indices of coronary disease is imperfect. Finally, lesion severity is often underestimated due to vessel remodeling or when the plaque is eccentric, and subjective assessment of stenosis severity at angiography introduces a further source of inaccuracy.

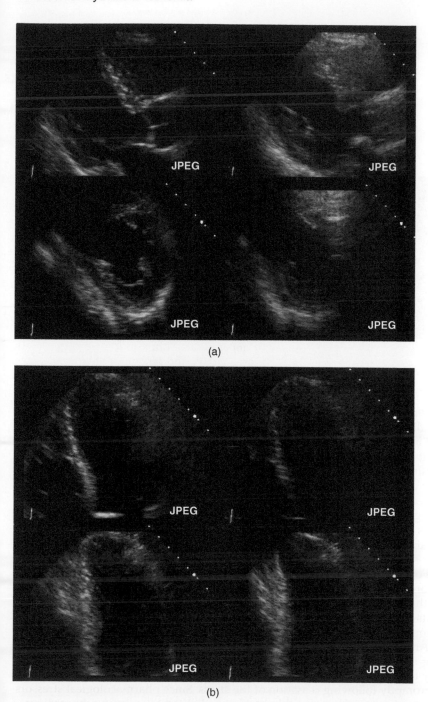

(a)

(b)

FIGURE 4 Implications of a negative stress echo. The identification of normal resting function (**A,B**) is an important precursor to the attribution of exertional dyspnea to increased filling pressure, evidenced by increased E/E′ (**C**) (loops 39 and 40).

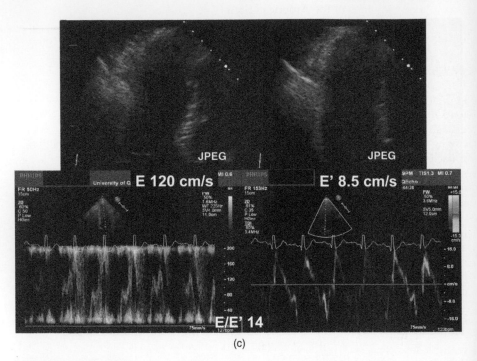

(c)

FIGURE 4 (*Continued*)

Adequacy of Stress

As the diagnosis of ischemia during stress echocardiography is based on recognition of inducible wall motion abnormalities, the ability of stress to ensure development of significant, sustained ischemia is one of the most important factors determining the accuracy of the test. As the increase in cardiac workload is greater with exercise than pharmacological stress, we consider exercise to be the preferred modality, as long as the patient is able to exercise maximally or pharmacological stress is not required for some other specific indication (e.g., simultaneous assessment of myocardial viability) (10,11). In contrast, in patients who are unable to exercise maximally, pharmacological stress imaging is preferred, as long as side effects do not limit dose.

For similar reasons, testing on antianginal therapy (especially β-blockers) may compromise the ability to provoke significant ischemia and thus adversely affect the sensitivity of the test. The addition of atropine may be helpful in such patients, but is often confined to pharmacological stress testing because of lack of venous access in patients undergoing exercise stress (12).

Another manifestation of the requirement to induce sufficient ischemia during stress echocardiography is the need to image the patient at or immediately after peak stress as the ischemic changes are transient and often disappear promptly following cessation of the stress. Since pharmacological stressors allow imaging at peak stress, this problem is limited to exercise echocardiography. Upright or supine bicycle ergometry have been shown to have higher sensitivity than treadmill stress echocardiography for the same reason (13). However, the ability to image at peak stress is counterbalanced by the technical difficulties of this as well as the lower workload achieved during cycle ergometry (14).

Echocardiographic Factors
Poor image quality may compromise the accuracy and reproducibility of the stress echocardiography, particularly for the assessment of the extent of the disease. Even in patients with reasonable image quality, there are regional differences. The basal segment of the inferior wall often appears to be hypokinetic owing to tethering to the plane of the mitral valve and shadowing by papillary muscles, causing poor endocardial definition. Similarly, interpretation of basal septum is compromised due to the membranous septum being visualized if the apical four-chamber view is angulated toward the aortic root. For these reasons, isolated wall motion abnormalities involving these segments without evidence of ischemia in adjacent segments are often misleading and a common cause for false-positive results. In contrast, the lateral wall is often a site for false negatives as the endocardium of the lateral wall, being parallel to the ultrasound beam, may not be very well visualized in the apical four-chamber view. The use of harmonic imaging, lateral gain correction, and LV opacification has reduced this problem (Fig. 5).

Finally, the influence of the skill and expertise of the interpreter in determining the results of the stress echocardiography has already been discussed. Adequate training, strict adherence to the systematic stepwise approach, joint reading sessions, and interpreting stress echocardiograms blinded to the clinical data are some of the ways to eliminate subjectivity and interpreter bias and are immensely helpful in improving the accuracy of results and the concordance among readers (2,5).

B. Accuracy of Exercise and Pharmacological Stress Echocardiography

Accuracy of Exercise Echocardiography
This has been examined in numerous studies, in studies of >100 patients, the sensitivity of exercise echocardiography has been shown to range from 74% to 97% with specificity being 64% to 86% (Fig. 6). In 44 studies of exercise echocardiography included in a recent meta-analysis, the average sensitivity and specificity were 83% and 84%, respectively (15). The angiographic cutoff of luminal diameter stenosis required to provoke inducible wall motion abnormalities at exercise echocardiography is 54%, with stenosis diameters of 0.7 to 1.0 mm by quantitative angiography (16,17). As expected, the sensitivity for detection of patients with single-vessel disease has been lower (59–94%) than those for detection of multivessel disease (85–100%), although the extent of ischemia is often underestimated in patients with multivessel disease (18–20).

Accuracy of Dobutamine Stress Echocardiography
In the studies enrolling >100 patients, sensitivity of dobutamine stress echocardiography has been shown to range between 61% and 96% with specificity ranging from 51% to 95% (Table 3). In the above meta-analysis, 80 studies of dobutamine echocardiography showed an average sensitivity of 80% and specificity of 85% for the detection of coronary artery disease (15). The addition of atropine has been known to increase the sensitivity of dobutamine echocardiography

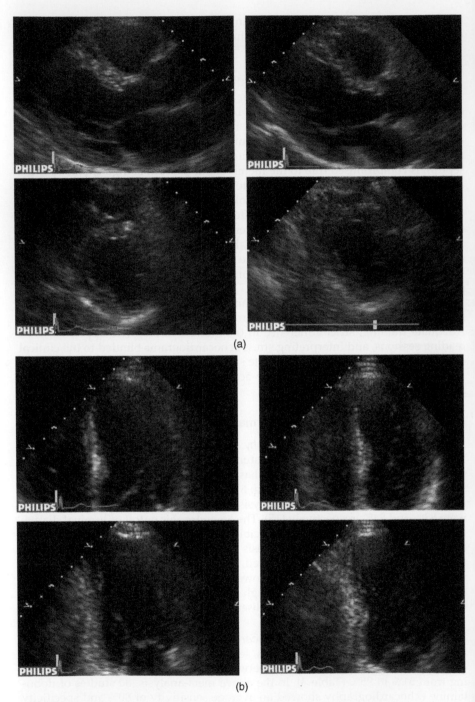

FIGURE 5 Role of LVO in detection of posterolateral ischemia. Standard 2-D images (**A,B**) were interpreted as normal. The use of LVO permits recognition of a posterolateral wall motion abnormality, corresponding to left circumflex disease.

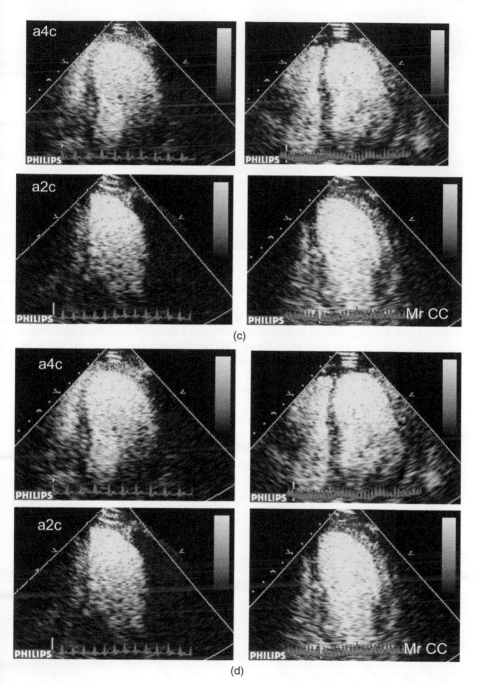

FIGURE 5 (Continued)

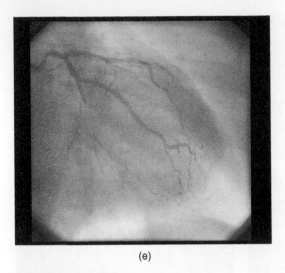

(e)

FIGURE 5 (*Continued*)

allowing attainment of target heart rate in greater proportion of patients (12). At quantitative angiography, a lumen diameter of <1 mm, percent diameter stenosis of 52%, and percent area stenosis of 75% have been shown to correlate with development of ischemia during dobutamine echocardiography with minimum lumen diameter being the most predictive (21). In addition, for obvious reasons, dobutamine echocardiography has been shown to be a more sensitive marker of ischemia in lesions involving larger (>2.6-mm diameter) vessels than smaller vessels (22). Similar to exercise echocardiography, the sensitivity of dobutamine echocardiography for detection of ischemia in patients with multivessel disease is higher than in those with single-vessel disease. However, the ability to predict multivessel disease itself varies depending on the patient subset being studied.

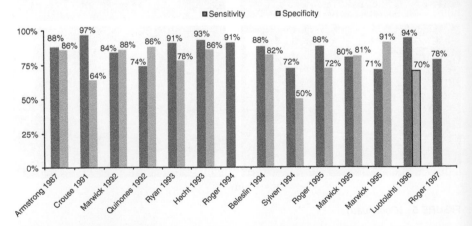

FIGURE 6 Accuracy of exercise echocardiography for detection of angiographic coronary artery disease, limited to studies with >100 patients.

TABLE 3 Accuracy of Dobutamine Stress Echocardiography for Detection of Angiographic Coronary Artery Disease, Limited to Studies with >100 Patients

Author (year)	Total no. of patients	Dobutamine protocol	Significant CAD (%)	Multivessel CAD (% all CAD)	Previous MI (% all CAD)	Sensitivity (%)	Sensitivity-SVD patients (%)	Specificity (%)
Sawada (71)	103	30 μg/kg/min	>50	41 (40)	35 (43)	95 ($n=81$)	89 ($n=38$)	77 ($n=22$)
Marcovitz (72)	141	30 μg/kg/min	>50	47 (43)	—	96 ($n=109$)	95 ($n=62$)	66 ($n=32$)
Marwick (73)	217	40 μg/kg/min	>50	74 (52)	0 (0)	72 ($n=142$)	66 ($n=68$)	83 ($n=75$)
Takeuchi (74)	120	30 μg/kg/min	>50	37 (50)	62 (84)	85 ($n=74$)	73 ($n=37$)	93 ($n=46$)
Beleslin (75)	136	40 μg/kg/min	>50	11 (9)	41 (34)	82 ($n=119$)	82 ($n=108$)	77 ($n=27$)
Ostojic (76)	150	40 μg/kg/min	>50	16 (12)	38 (29)	75 ($n=131$)	—	79 ($n=19$)
Pingitore (77)	110	40 μg/kg/min + atropine	>50	42 (46)	25 (27)	84 ($n=92$)	—	89 ($n=18$)
Ling (78)	183	40 μg/kg/min + atropine	>70	109 (74)	105 (71)	95 ($n=148$)	—	51 ($n=35$)
San Roman (79)	102	40 μg/kg/min + atropine	>50	34 (54)	0 (0)	77 ($n=63$)	68 ($n=29$)	95 ($n=39$)
Anthopoulos (80)	120	40 μg/kg/min + atropine	>50	48 (40)	38 (30)	87 ($n=89$)	74 ($n=19$)	84 ($n=31$)
Dionisopoulos (81)	288	40 μg/kg/min + atropine	>50	122 (58)	—	87 ($n=209$)	80 ($n=70$)	89 ($n=79$)
Elhendy (82)	96 f, 210 m	40 μg/kg/min + atropine	>50	142 (61)	214 (70)	76 ($n=62$), 73 ($n=171$)	64, 56	94 ($n=34$), 77 ($n=39$)
Hennessy (83)	219	40 μg/kg/min + atropine	>50	113 (66)	55 (24)	82 ($n=170$)	74 ($n=57$)	65 ($n=49$)
Nagel (84)	208	40 μg/kg/min + atropine	>50	70 (64)	0 (0)	74 ($n=107$)	67 ($n=39$)	70 ($n=101$)
Beleslin (85)	168	40 μg/kg/min	>50	0 (0)	40 (24)	61 ($n=153$)	61 ($n=153$)	88 ($n=25$)

Abbreviations: CAD, coronary artery disease; MI, myocardial infarction; SVD, single-vessel disease; TEE, transesophageal echocardiography.
Source: From Ref. 61.

The sensitivity is higher (80–85%) in patients with a history of previous myocardial infarction, as compared to the patients without previous infarction (approximately 50%).

Accuracy of Vasodilator Stress Echocardiography
Significant studies of >50 patients have shown the sensitivity and specificity of dipyridamole and adenosine stress echocardiography for the detection of coronary artery disease to range between 61–96% and 90–96%, respectively (Table 4). In the meta-analysis described earlier, 40 studies of dipyridamole and 11 studies of adenosine echocardiography were included which showed an average sensitivity of 71% and a specificity of 92% for dipyridamole and 68% and 81%, respectively, for adenosine (15). Again, the addition of atropine tends to increase the sensitivity of these techniques by adding the element of increased myocardial oxygen demand to the decreased blood supply induced by the vasodilator (23). At quantitative angiography, parameters that have been shown to predict an abnormal dipyridamole echocardiogram include a stenotic flow reserve of <2.8, stenosis diameter >59%, lumen diameter <1.35 mm, and coronary flow reserve <2.0 (24). Other studies have confirmed that the optimal angiographic cutoff for dipyridamole stress echocardiography is 60%, as compared with 58% for dobutamine and 54% for exercise echocardiography (17).

Accuracy of Pacing Stress Echocardiography
In the meta-analysis referred to earlier, 23 studies of atrial-pacing stress echocardiography (16 using transesophageal and 7 using transthoracic echocardiography) were included. Mean sensitivity and specificity for pacing combined with transesophageal imaging were 86% and 91%, respectively, and were 91% and 86%, respectively, for transthoracic imaging (15). These favorable results probably reflect the combination of high-quality images obtained with transesophageal imaging and the ability to reach target heart rate reproducibly using atrial pacing. However, the invasive nature and the technical complexity of the test have limited its widespread use compared to other forms of stress echocardiography.

IV. SELECTION OF OPTIMAL STRESSOR

A. Exercise Vs. Pharmacological Stress
In patients who are able to perform maximal exercise, exercise stress is associated with numerous advantages and is generally the preferred mode of stress testing. Exercise provides a greater level of stress on heart as both the heart rate and the blood pressure (and thus the rate-pressure product) increase with increasing workload (10,11). In contrast, heart rate increases with increasing dobutamine dose, but the blood pressure response is variable. The ability to induce ischemia is therefore greater with exercise stress and this compensates for the problems associated with delay in imaging poststress and the influence of respiratory motion on the quality of imaging. Markers of severe disease (e.g., LV cavity dilatation, reduction in ejection fraction) are more likely with exercise compared to dobutamine as the afterload lowering effect of latter counterbalances the tendency of ischemia to increase LV cavity size (7).

Exercise also provides other valuable information, which may not be available with pharmacological stress testing. This includes ST-segment changes and

TABLE 4 Accuracy of Vasodilator (Dipyridamole and Adenosine) Echocardiography for Detection of Angiographic Coronary Artery Disease, Limited to Studies with >100 Patients

Author (year)	Total no. of patients	Stress protocol	Significant CAD (%)	Multivessel CAD (% all CAD)	Previous MI (% all CAD)	Sensitivity (%)	Specificity (%)
Picano (86)	445	Dipy 0.84 mg/kg[a]	>50	119 (46)	0 (0)	96 (n = 256)	96
Severi (87)	429	Dipy 0.84 mg/kg[a]	>75	114 (46)	0	75 (n = 246)	90
Picano (88)	130	Dipy 0.84 mg/kg + atropine[a]	>50	—	—	87 (n = 94)	94
Ostojic (76)	150	Dipy 0.84 mg/kg[a]	>50	16 (12)	38 (29)	71 (n = 131)	89
Beleslin (75)	136	Dipy 0.84 mg/kg[a]	>50	11 (9)	41(34)	74 (n = 119)	94 (n = 17)
San Roman (79)	102	Dipy 0.84 mg/kg[a]	>50	34 (54)	0 (0)	77 (n = 63)	97
Pingitore (77)	110	Dipy 0.84 mg/kg + atropine[a]	>50			82 (n = 92)	94
Anthopoulos (80)	120	Ad 0.14 mg/kg/min[a]	>50	48 (40)	38 (30)	66 (n = 89)	90 (n = 31)
Beleslin (85)	168	Dipy 0.84 mg/kg[a]	>50	0 (0)	40 (24)	61 (n = 153)	88 (n = 25)

[a] Low-dose positivity permits conclusion of study before stated "peak" dose.
Abbreviations: Ad, adenosine; CAD, coronary artery disease; Dipy, dipyridamole; MI, myocardial infarction.
Source: From Ref. 61.

maximal exercise capacity (important prognostic markers), correlation of symptoms with activity level, cardiac hemodynamics with stress (contractile reserve, systemic, and pulmonary artery pressure), etc.

In patients who are unable to exercise maximally, pharmacological stress testing is clearly the first choice. Other than this, pharmacological stress testing has its own advantages. These include better image quality (as the patient is stationary and there is not much tachypnea), ability to image the heart at both low-level and peak stress and the relative ease with which it can be combined with newer techniques such as deformation analysis and contrast echocardiography. Imaging during stepwise increments of stress allows estimation of ischemic threshold which can not only be helpful in predicting the extent of disease but is a valuable prognostic marker also (25,26). The identification of myocardial viability, which requires an assessment of myocardial response to low-level stress, is best performed with pharmacological stress and may be reason to perform dobutamine rather than exercise echocardiography in a patient who is able to exercise. Furthermore, augmentation of contractility at low dose facilitates identification of ischemia at higher dose and therefore pharmacological stress testing is particularly useful in patients with previous myocardial infarction and resting wall motion abnormalities (27).

The accuracy of both exercise and pharmacological stress testing has been compared in several studies by performing both the tests in the same patients (Table 5). The results of these studies suggest that both the techniques to have similar diagnostic accuracy for detection of coronary artery disease and therefore the choice between the two is based on factors other than diagnostic accuracy as described above.

B. Selection of the Optimal Nonexercise Stress

Studies based on head-to-head comparison between dobutamine and vasodilator stress have generally demonstrated higher sensitivity of dobutamine for detection of coronary artery disease (Table 6)—driven mainly by superiority of dobutamine for detection of single-vessel disease. This gives dobutamine a slight advantage as a diagnostic test for CAD in the symptomatic patient. In contrast, both dobutamine and dipyridamole have similar efficacy for prognostic assessment (28). The additional factors that guide this selection include the presence or absence of specific contraindications to the use of particular agent (e.g., vasodilators are preferable in patients with hypertension or arrhythmias, and dobutamine is better with significant conduction disturbances or asthma), as well as local experience and cost. In contrast, atrial-pacing echocardiography remains largely underutilized apart from in patients with permanently implanted pacemaker. It does offer a viable alternative to other forms of stress testing in patients in whom target heart rate cannot be achieved due to intrinsic conduction system abnormality.

V. COMPARISON WITH OTHER TECHNIQUES

Numerous studies and meta-analyses have attempted to compare the diagnostic accuracy of the stress echocardiography with other forms of stress testing in a wide variety of patient subsets. The studies that have compared different techniques directly in the same patients are generally preferable, although they overcome some but not most of these problems.

TABLE 5 Sensitivity and Specificity of Exercise and Nonexercise Stress Echocardiography in >50 Patients

Author (year)	Significant CAD (%)	Multivessel CAD (% all CAD)	Previous MI (% all CAD)	CAD patients	Sensitivity (%)				No CAD patients	Specificity (%)				Comments
					Ex	Db	Dipy	TAP		Ex	Db	Dipy	TAP	
Picano (89)	>70	18 (53)	6 (18)	34	76	—	72	—	21	81	—	100	—	Ex and dipy comparable
Hoffman (90)	>70	21 (42)	0 (0)	50	80	79	—	—	16	87	81	—	—	Ex and Db comparable
Cohen (91)	>70	21 (57)	11 (30)	37	78	86	—	—	15	87	87	—	—	Ex and Db comparable
Beleslin (75)	>50	11 (9)	41 (34)	119	80	82	74	—	17	82	77	94	—	Ex, Db, and dipy comparable
Marangelli (92)	>75	19 (54)	—	35	89	—	43	83	25	91	—	92	76	Ex has best balance of sensitivity & specificity
Marwick (93)	>50	34 (61)	0 (0)	56	88	54	—	—	30	80	83	—	—	Ex superior with submaximal Db
Dagianti (94)	>70	15 (60)	0 (0)	25	76	72	52	—	35	94	97	97	—	Ex and Db comparable, dipy inferior
San Roman (79)	>50	34 (54)	0 (0)	63	68	77	77	—	39	79	95	97	—	Ex less specific, sensitivity same
Kisacik (95)	>50	—	—	47	57	90	—	—	22	62	90	—	—	Db superior
Rallidis (96)	>70	40 (47)	42 (49)	85	73	62	—	—	0	—	—	—	—	Only known CAD; Ex may be preferable
Santoro (97)	>70	21 (64)	0 (0)	33	58	61	55	—	27	67	96	96	—	Ex less reliable

Abbreviations: CAD, coronary artery disease; Db, dobutamine; Dipy, dipyridamole; Ex, exercise; MI, myocardial infarction; SVD, single-vessel disease; TAP, atrial pacing.
Sources: From Refs. 20, 61–63.

TABLE 6 Studies Comparing Sensitivity and Specificity of Dobutamine and Vasodilator Stress Echocardiography in >50 Patients

Author (year)	Total no. of patients	Vasodilator	CAD patients (% all)	Multivessel CAD (% all CAD)	Previous MI (% all CAD)	Sensitivity (%)		Specificity (%)	
						Dobutamine	Vasodilator	Dobutamine	Vasodilator
Marwick (98)	97	Adenosine	59 (61)	28 (47)	0 (0)	85	58	82	87
Previtali (99)	80	Dipyridamole	57 (71)	33 (58)	15 (26)	79	60	83	96
Beleslin (75)	136	Dipyridamole	119 (88)	11 (9)	41(34)	82	74	77	94
Ostojic (76)	150	Dipyridamole	131 (87)	16 (12)	38 (29)	75	71	79	89
Dagianti (94)	60	Dipyridamole	25 (42)	15 (60)	41 (39)	72	52	97	97
San Roman (79)	102	Dipyridamole	63 (62)	34 (54)	0 (0)	77	77	95	97
Anthopoulos (80)	120	Adenosine	89 (74)	48 (40)	38 (30)	87	66	84	90
Santoro (97)	60	Dipyridamole	33 (55)	21 (64)	0 (0)	61	55	96	96
Loimaala (100)	60	Dipyridamole	44 (73)	18 (41)	0 (0)	93	95	63	75
Fragasso (101)	101	Dipyridamole	56 (56)	37 (65)	0 (0)	88	61	80	91

Abbreviations: CAD, coronary artery disease; MI, myocardial infarction.
Sources: From Refs. 20, 61.

A. Comparison with Stress Electrocardiography

Stress ECG is the oldest, simplest, and the most widely used stress-testing modality. However, this test has limited applicability in two major scenarios: patients who are unable to perform maximal exercise and those with uninterpretable ECG, accounting for more than half of the patients undergoing stress testing at many tertiary referral centers. As a result, previous studies have shown significant variability in the accuracy of this test, with overall sensitivity and specificity in the range of 70%. Even in patients who are able to exercise maximally and who have interpretable ECG, sensitivity and specificity of stress ECG are inferior to that of stress echocardiography (29). The higher sensitivity of stress echocardiography may reflect the fact that development of wall motion abnormalities precedes development of ECG changes or chest pain in the ischemic cascade (30). The better specificity of the stress echocardiography is a manifestation of the fact that inducible regional wall motion abnormalities are rarely caused by anything other than ischemia, whereas ECG changes may be due to other conditions. These differences may lead to superior cost-effectiveness for exercise echocardiography because potential false-positive and -negative stress results are often investigated further (Fig. 7). Nevertheless, despite the aforementioned

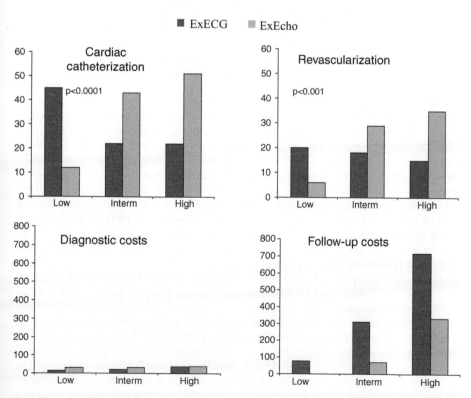

FIGURE 7 Catheterization, revascularization, and costs of ExECG (purple) and ExE (blue). Catheterization was performed in a disproportionate number of low-probability patients studied by ExECG, likely reflecting reluctance of clinicians to rely on these data due to limitations in accuracy. Angiographic findings drive revascularization such that the minor increment of diagnostic costs with stress echo is dwarfed by follow-up costs.

inadequacies of the stress ECG, its wholesale replacement with stress echocardiography as the initial diagnostic test would not be feasible and not recommended at present. However, there are certain specific patient subsets in whom stress ECG is less reliable and therefore stress imaging might be considered as the initial diagnostic test in spite of an interpretable ECG and the patient's ability to achieve adequate workload. These include women, patients with hypertensive heart disease, and patients with previous revascularization.

Although most diagnostic tests used for detection of coronary artery disease have when applied in women, exercise ECG appears to be the worst affected of all (31). Lower pretest probability of disease in women, less extensive disease, inability to perform maximal exercise, and poor reliability of ST changes are all the reasons for suboptimal accuracy of stress ECG in women. In contrast, the accuracy of stress echocardiography is affected to a much lesser degree in women and several studies have consistently shown it to have higher sensitivity and specificity than stress ECG (32). Moreover, stress echocardiography has also been shown to be cost-effective as the initial diagnostic test in women, the benefit driven primarily by its significantly higher specificity resulting in substantial reduction in the performance of unwarranted angiograms (32).

Another subset of patients in whom noninvasive detection of coronary artery disease is really challenging are individuals with left ventricular hypertrophy. Nonspecific ST-T changes are common during exercise in these patients and significantly compromise the specificity of stress ECG. In contrast, stress echocardiography once again has been shown to be more accurate and cost-effective means of identifying coronary artery disease in these patients (33).

B. Comparison with Stress Perfusion Imaging

Myocardial perfusion scintigraphy is the main alternative to stress echocardiography for both the detection of ischemia and the assessment of myocardial viability (the two major indications for stress imaging) and hence the two techniques are considered to be the direct competitors. Studies dealing with individual techniques have generally shown perfusion scintigraphy to have higher sensitivity (>90%) and lower sensitivity (approximately 70%) than that reported for stress echocardiography for the detection of coronary artery disease but the overall accuracy has been comparable. In a meta-analysis including 44 studies using stress echocardiography and/or stress perfusion scintigraphy for detection of coronary artery disease, Fleischmann et al. reported the average sensitivity and specificity of stress echocardiography to be 85% and 77% and that of perfusion scintigraphy to be 87% and 64%, respectively (34). When adjusted for age, publication year, and known coronary artery disease, stress echocardiography had better discriminatory power than SPECT. However, several technical issues related to the differences in the tracer, reading protocols, and gating could have affected the diagnostic accuracy of SPECT in this meta-analysis and moreover, this analysis did not include the studies involving pharmacological stress. A review of the studies that have directly compared the two techniques in the same patients using a variety of stressors shows somewhat higher sensitivity but lower specificity of perfusion scintigraphy, but the differences were not statistically significant (Table 7). Thus there is nothing much to choose between the two techniques in terms of diagnostic accuracy and several additional factors need to be taken in to consideration before making selection between one of

TABLE 7 Head-to-Head Comparisons of Stress Echocardiography and Myocardial Perfusion Imaging in >50 Patients

Author (year)	Total no. of patients	Significant) CAD (%)	CAD patients	MVD (% all CAD)	Stress method	Nuclear method	Sensitivity (%) Echo	Sensitivity (%) Nuclear	Sensitivity (%) – SVD patients Echo	Sensitivity (%) – SVD patients Nuclear	Specificity (%) Echo	Specificity (%) Nuclear
Pozzoli (102)	75	>50	49	16 (33)	Upright bike	SPECT-MIBI	71	84	60	82	96	88
Galanti (103)	53	>50	27	14 (52)	Upright bike	Planar Tl	93	100	93	100	96	92
Quinones (104)	112	>50	86	45 (52)	Treadmill	SPECT-Tl	74	76	58	61	88	81
Hecht (105)	71	>50	51	29 (57)	Supine bike	SPECT-Tl	90	92	77	95	80	65
Marwick (98)	97	>50	59	28 (47)	Ad 0.84 mg/kg	SPECT-MIBI	58	86	—	—	87	71
					Db 40	—	85	80	—	—	82	74
Marwick (73)	217	>50	142	74 (52)	Db 40	SPECT-MIBI	72	76	66	74	83	67
Takeuchi (74)	120	>50	74	37 (50)	Db 30	SPECT-Tl	85	89	—	—	93	85
Senior (106)	61	>50	44	30 (68)	Db 40	SPECT-MIBI	93	95	86	86	94	71
Ho (107)	54	>50	43	—	Db 40	SPECT-Tl	93	98	—	—	73	73
San Roman (108)	72	>50	49	—	Db 40 + atropine	SPECT-MIBI	78	87	—	—	88	70
Kisacik (95)	69	>50	47	—	Treadmill	(treadmill only)	57	96	—	—	62	71
					Db 40	SPECT-Tl	90	—	—	—	90	—
Huang (109)	93	>50	67	—	Db 40	SPECT-Tl	93	90	—	—	77	81
Parodi (110)	101	≥50	80	43 (54)	Dipy 0.84 mg/kg	Planar Tl	78	79	—	—	76	90
Santoro (97)	60	>70	33	21 (64)	Db 40	SPECT-MIBI	61	91	—	—	96	81
Smart (111)	183	>50	119	58 (49)	Dipy 0.84 mg/kg	SPECT-MIBI	55	97	—	—	96	89
					Db 40 + atropine		87	80	84	71	91	73

Abbreviations: Ad, adenosine; CAD, coronary artery disease; Db, dobutamine; Dipy, dipyridamole; MIBI, Technetium-99m sestamibi; MVD, multivessel disease; SVD, single-vessel disease; Tl, thallium-201 chloride.
Sources: From Refs. 39, 61, 63–70.

these two modalities for diagnosis of coronary artery disease in the individual patients:

(a) *Local expertise*: Accuracy of both stress echocardiography and perfusion imaging is heavily dependent on the technical expertise of the interpreter and the quality and standard of the laboratory available. Although the need of expertise is greater for stress echocardiography, the role of quantification in SPECT imaging may be overstated and the technique still requires an expert eye. Therefore, the most important factor determining the choice between the tests should always be the level of expertise at the local imaging facility. The centers with excellence in nuclear should preferably opt for nuclear imaging while the converse is true for the centers with excellence in stress echocardiography. Only when the comparable expertise exists for both the modalities, should other factors be taken into consideration.

(b) *Dependence on image quality*: Image quality plays an important role in determining the accuracy and the reproducibility of the stress echocardiography results and remains an important limitation of the technique despite technical advances such as digital processing, side-by-side display of the cine loops, and harmonic imaging. Clear visualization of the endocardium and reproduction of the same imaging planes during the different stages of stress testing are essential to ensure accurate interpretation. Because of a variety of reasons including obesity, pulmonary disease, and chest deformities, optimal-quality images are acquired in perhaps 70% of the patients undergoing stress echocardiography. If LV opacification is not available, perfusion scintigraphy is a superior modality in such patients.

(c) *Induction of ischemia versus perfusion mismatch*: As discussed earlier, stress echocardiography relies on identification of wall motion abnormalities, which develop at a later stage in the ischemic cascade than the abnormalities of perfusion (30). Therefore, perfusion scintigraphy has better sensitivity for detection of the coronary artery disease than stress echocardiography and the discrepancy is greater when the extent and/or severity of the disease are milder. Thus perfusion scintigraphy tends to be more accurate in patients with single-vessel disease, mild stenoses, and in those who are on antianginal therapy (35–37). Furthermore, for the same reason, stress echocardiography is more likely to underestimate the extent of coronary artery disease than perfusion scintigraphy which appears to be significantly more sensitive for the recognition of multivessel disease (38). This difference can be reversed by using echo contrast agents to assess perfusion (Fig. 8).

(d) *Site of disease*: Several factors adversely influence the ability of stress echocardiography to localize the site of disease accurately. These include difficulties in evaluation of inferior and lateral walls due to the reasons already described and the ambiguity in allocation of myocardial segments to different coronary vascular territories. In a review of 10 published studies enrolling 970 patients, O'Keefe et al. demonstrated a nonsignificant trend toward better localization of coronary disease with exercise perfusion scintigraphy compared to exercise echocardiography (sensitivity 79% vs. 65%). However, for detection of left circumflex disease, the sensitivity of exercise echocardiography was substantially worse than perfusion imaging (33% vs. 72%, $p < 0.001$), although it should be recognized that these were older studies without harmonics or LV opacification (38).

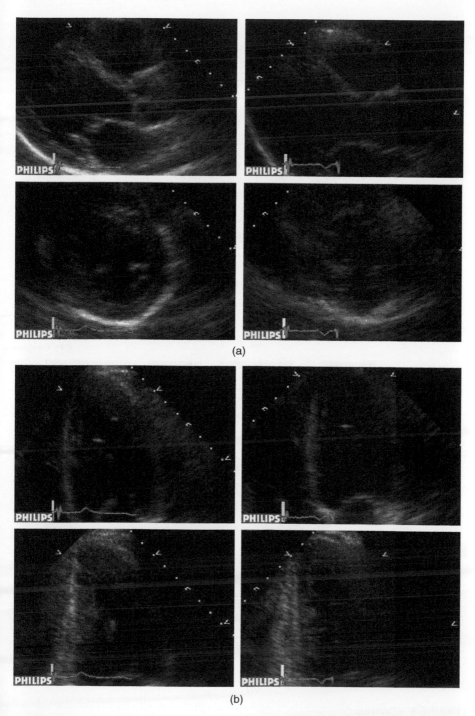

FIGURE 8 Incremental value of MCE for disease extent. Standard 2-D images (**A,B**) show borderline abnormalities. Destruction–replenishment images show inferior and apical subendo-cardial defects (**C,D**), corresponding to multivessel CAD (**E**) (loops 41 and 42).

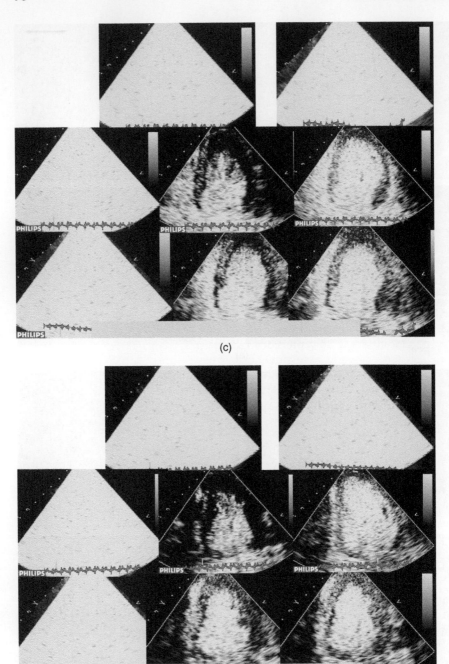

(c)

(d)

FIGURE 8 (*Continued*)

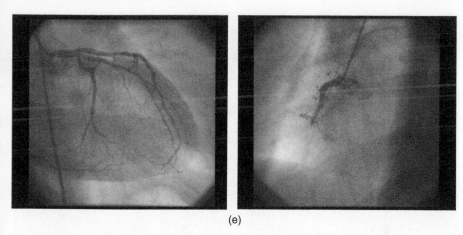

(e)

FIGURE 8 (*Continued*)

(e) *Resting wall motion abnormalities*: Recognition of ischemia on stress echocar-diography is usually difficult in patients with resting wall motion abnor-malities because of the difficulty in accurate identification of minor differ-ences in the severity of regional dysfunction. Hence perfusion scintigraphy appears to be superior to the stress echocardiography in this setting (39).

(f) *Women*: As already discussed, accurate detection of coronary artery disease noninvasively is technically challenging in women due to a variety of rea-sons. Of all the available modalities, stress echocardiography appears to be the best in this situation. Relatively poor spatial resolution (considering the smaller heart size) and problems related to breast tissue attenuation are the major disadvantages of the perfusion scintigraphy in this setting (40).

(g) *Left ventricular hypertrophy*: The presence of left ventricular hypertrophy is usually associated with microvascular abnormalities, which can result in false-positive results on perfusion scintigraphy (41). On the other hand, false-negative studies are also common due to reduction in coronary flow reserve which compromises ability to detect reversible defects on perfu-sion scintigraphy. Stress echocardiography is not significantly influenced by these abnormalities and thus appears to be the most accurate test in this setting (41). However, when left ventricular hypertrophy is associated with reduced LV cavity size (which is not uncommon), the likelihood of false-negative stress echocardiography increases. The underlying reasons for this include reduced wall stress with smaller cavity size and difficulty in recog-nition of wall motion abnormalities over smaller endocardial circumference (Fig. 9).

(h) *Left bundle-branch block*: Similar to left ventricular hypertrophy, left bundle-branch block (LBBB) is also known to commonly produce reversible or fixed perfusion defects on exercise stress scintigraphy in the absence of CAD (42). False-positive perfusion abnormalities are less common on vasodilator stress perfusion imaging, because although diastole is delayed due to the conduction abnormality, the tachycardia-induced shortening of diastole is avoided in vasodilator stress (42). Stress echocardiography has also proved to be a useful technique in patients with LBBB. In a recently published

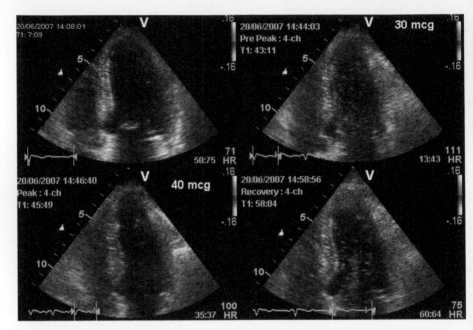

FIGURE 9 LV cavity size and accuracy of dobutamine stress echo. Progressive reduction of LV size during stress may compromise the sensitivity of DSE (loop 43).

meta-analysis, Biagini compared the diagnostic accuracy of stress ECG (6 studies), stress perfusion imaging (43 studies), and stress echocardiography (6 studies) in patients with left bundle-branch block (43). As compared to stress echocardiography, stress ECG and perfusion imaging had a higher sensitivity (75%, 83%, and 82% respectively) but much lower specificity (89%, 60%, and 41% respectively) and overall diagnostic accuracy (84%, 66%, and 70% respectively). Although the specificity of perfusion imaging improved dramatically with the use of pharmacological stress (from 23% with exercise stress to 74% with pharmacological stress), it was still inferior to that of pharmacological stress echocardiography.

(i) *Other factors*: Stress echocardiography has several additional practical advantages. It is readily available, patient friendly, and inexpensive and does not involve radiation exposure to the patient or environment. Moreover, when needed, echocardiography can provide a vast range of valuable information about other cardiac structures (e.g., valves, pericardium), function, and hemodynamics, which is not available from nuclear imaging. In fact, when stress testing is needed in patients with another cardiac disease (such as aortic stenosis, mitral regurgitation, and hypertrophic cardiomyopathy), the selection of stress echocardiography minimizes the number of tests required.

VI. NEW TECHNOLOGIES AND STRESS ECHOCARDIOGRAPHY

As discussed earlier, dependence on image quality and subjective interpretation significantly influence the feasibility, diagnostic accuracy, and reproducibility of stress echocardiography and remain the two major limitations of the technique.

Further advancements are certainly needed to overcome these issues and two relatively newer echocardiographic techniques, myocardial imaging and contrast echocardiography, appear particularly promising in this context. While myocardial imaging primarily addresses the issue of subjective interpretation, contrast permits the performance of LV opacification (a solution to the problem of image quality), as well as myocardial contrast (MCE). Allowing the recognition of subtle abnormalities of contractile function (myocardial imaging) or simultaneous assessment of myocardial perfusion (MCE) offers the potential to render stress echocardiography more sensitive for detection of myocardial ischemia.

A. Myocardial Imaging for Quantitation During Stress Echocardiography

The various quantitative techniques that have been developed for the quantitation of stress echocardiography can be categorized broadly into two groups—those based on measurement of endocardial motion from two-dimensional images (e.g., standard and anatomic M-mode, acoustic quantification, and color kinesis) and those based on measurement of myocardial velocity and strain. Although the initial studies with M-mode and color kinesis showed some promise, their dependence on very good image quality and sensitivity to the influences of translational movement of the heart have greatly limited their widespread use. In contrast, recently developed tissue-Doppler techniques have several advantages over the previous ones and appear to be the future of quantitative stress echocardiography.

In studies employing SPECT or angiographic correlation, peak systolic myocardial velocity has been shown to be moderately accurate for the recognition of ischemia during stress echocardiography (44,45). Nonetheless, it reflects movement of myocardium relative to the transducer, which can result from tethering by adjacent segments or translational cardiac motion. Strain and strain rate, unlike myocardial tissue velocity, are measures of deformation of myocardium and therefore reflect true myocardial motion and are not affected by tethering or translational movements. Strain rate is the rate of deformation—an analog of dP/dt—and is derived by calculating the instantaneous difference in myocardial velocity at two different points. Strain measures the extent of deformation—a marker of regional EF—and is calculated by integration of strain rate over time.

When applied to stress echocardiography, the attained peak systolic strain rate and presence of postsystolic shortening have been shown to be the features that are most predictive of ischemia (46,47). In a recent study in 197 patients undergoing dobutamine stress echocardiography, automated measurement of peak strain rate at peak stress was shown to have significantly higher sensitivity for detection of angiographic coronary artery disease compared to wall motion analysis alone by an expert reader. The specificity and overall accuracy were also higher for strain rate measurements, although the difference was not significant (48). Yet another study involving 646 patients undergoing dobutamine stress echocardiography revealed peak strain rate measured using automated analysis to provide prognostic information that was independent and incremental to standard wall motion score index (49). In contrast, Voigt et al. found postsystolic shortening measured using strain analysis to be the most accurate marker of ischemia (46). At the least, deformation analysis can be used as an adjunct to facilitate the assessment of difficult studies (Fig. 10).

Despite these favorable results, strain rate imaging also has several limitations to its routine application during stress echocardiography. It is technically

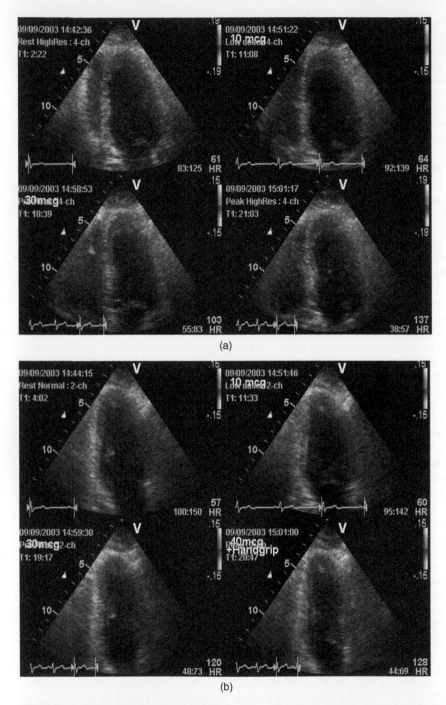

FIGURE 10 Use of strain rate imaging to confirm wall motion analysis. Standard 2-D images (**A,B**) show questionable inferior wall motion abnormalities. Deformation analysis (**C,D**) shows reduction and delay of basal septal and inferior deformation, confirming RCA disease (**E**).

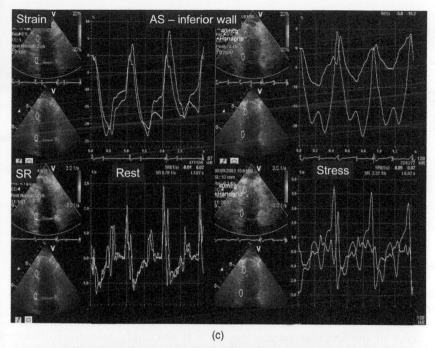

(c)

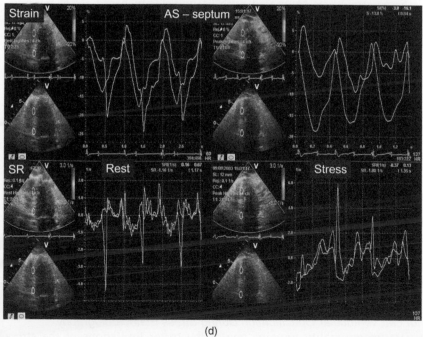

(d)

FIGURE 10 (*Continued*)

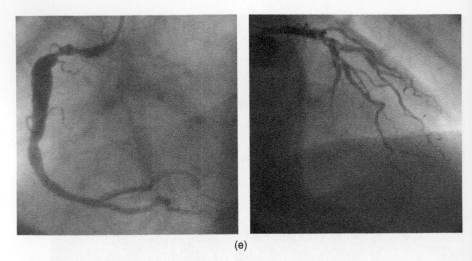

(e)

FIGURE 10   (*Continued*)

challenging, has significant signal noise, and, the most importantly, is heavily dependent on insonation angle. Recently two-dimensional strain measurement techniques have been developed for overcoming issues related to angle-dependence of the Doppler parameters. In a recent study, two-dimensional, speckle-based strain was compared with tissue velocity–based strain parameters for detection of angiographically significant coronary artery disease during stress echocardiography (50). The diagnostic accuracy of these strain parameters were found to be similar but not superior to wall motion analysis by an expert reader. The two techniques had comparable accuracy for detection of ischemia in the anterior circulation but tissue velocity–based measures were found to be superior to the corresponding two-dimensional strain parameters for detection of ischemia in the posterior circulation. This discrepancy probably reflects the dependence of speckle-based strain on image quality.

B.   Myocardial Contrast Echocardiography

The use of contrast agents offers two major advantages over conventional echocardiographic imaging—LV cavity opacification (resulting in improved delineation of endocardial border) and the ability to assess regional myocardial perfusion. Both these characteristics of the contrast imaging are of particular benefit during stress echocardiography and several studies have now demonstrated improvement in the diagnostic accuracy of stress echocardiography with the use of contrast imaging (51). In addition, pharmacoeconomic analyses have indicated contrast imaging during stress echocardiography to be cost-effective because of savings in subsequent investigations despite the initial expenditure involved in the use of contrast agents (52).

MCE for Left Ventricular Opacification During Stress Echocardiography

Inadequate image quality remains one of the major limitations of the stress echocardiography and significantly influences the accuracy of the test. In patients with poor-quality images, interinstitutional agreement for the interpretation of results has been reported to be as low as 43% (53). Failure to perform a good-quality complete study may occur in up to 30% of the patients undergoing stress echocardiography, even with the use of the latest imaging techniques. The use of the contrast imaging for LV opacification may overcome this limitation (51,54–56). In a study on 300 patients, Rainbird et al. demonstrated significant improvement in the wall segment visualization and image quality at rest and at peak stress, resulting in improved confidence of interpretation (54). Numerous other studies have reported the benefits of LV cavity opacification in improving the image quality and salvaging otherwise uninterpretable studies (55,56). However, the influence of improved endocardial definition with LV cavity opacification on the diagnostic accuracy of stress echocardiography has been reported in a few studies only (57). Dolan et al. performed dobutamine stress echocardiography in 112 patients with good-quality images and 117 patients with poor-quality images at rest. Using contrast imaging in patients with poor-quality rest images, the sensitivity and specificity of the wall motion analysis for diagnosis of coronary artery disease were found to be 78% and 76%, respectively, which were remarkably comparable to the values obtained with standard imaging in those with good-quality rest images (71% and 82% respectively) (57).

MCE for Assessment of Myocardial Perfusion During Stress Echocardiograph

Using the intravenous contrast agents in combination with bubble destruction-replenishment techniques, regional myocardial blood flow can be reliably estimated both at rest and at peak stress. Assessment of myocardial perfusion with these techniques can be accomplished using both qualitative and quantitative methods. The former of these involves visual assessment of the speed and the extent of contrast filling in different myocardial segments whereas the latter requires mathematical computations based on the rate of increase in myocardial video intensity following bubble destruction. It was hoped that the use of quantitation would help reduce the subjectivity associated with qualitative assessment, thereby improving the accuracy and reproducibility of the results, but the technique remains technically challenging.

Initial studies comparing qualitative assessment of myocardial perfusion with MCE against nuclear imaging showed good agreement between the two techniques for detection of the perfusion defects and the concordance was better when wall motion analysis was combined with the perfusion data (58). More recent studies have employed coronary angiography as the gold standard to determine the diagnostic accuracy of myocardial contrast imaging (59). In a study on 85 patients, the addition of contrast (for LV opacification and perfusion assessment) to standard exercise echocardiography was shown to result in significant improvement in the sensitivity of the test for detection of coronary artery disease (from 74% to 91%) with a nonsignificant reduction in specificity (60). A pooled analysis of eight other such studies has revealed the sensitivity and specificity of MCE for detection of coronary artery disease to be 85% and 74%, respectively, compared to 71% and 71% for the standard stress echocardiography/SPECT tests (59).

Selection of optimal stressor for use in conjunction with myocardial contrast imaging is debatable at present. Although adenosine has the advantage of provoking the most intense and most predictive coronary hyperemia, the current evidence base is seriously limited in addressing this issue. Finally, while the value of LVO in technically difficult images is unquestionable, the cost-effectiveness of routine MCE during stress remains unclear. Moir et al. reported a comparison of noncontrast and contrast images showing an improvement in sensitivity with a minor decrement of accuracy (60). However, the anticipated prognostic benefits of increased sensitivity are small (because most coronary disease that is missed by wall motion analysis involves mild disease), so to make the addition of contrast cost-effective, the technique would need to improve specificity or be available at lower cost.

VII. CONCLUSIONS

The use of wall motion analysis in combination with stress has been shown to be an accurate means of detecting ischemia over many years. However, wall motion analysis requires training and has limitations in particular circumstances. The clinical application of new technologies such as myocardial imaging and contrast echocardiography will be part of the continued evolution of stress echocardiography into the future.

DVD note: The following loops are related to the content of this chapter: 6, 7, 19, 32–43, 82b–c, 85. These loops can be found in the provided DVD.

REFERENCES

1. Picano E, Lattanzi F, Orlandini A, et al. Stress echocardiography and the human factor: The importance of being expert. J Am Coll Cardiol 1991; 17:666–669.
2. Varga A, Picano E, Dodi C, et al. Madness and method in stress echo reading. Eur Heart J 1999; 20:1271–1275.
3. Hoffmann R, Lethen H, Marwick T, et al. Analysis of interinstitutional observer agreement in interpretation of dobutamine stress echocardiograms. J Am Coll Cardiol 1996; 27:330–336.
4. Hoffmann R, Marwick TH, Poldermans D, et al. Refinements in stress echocardiographic techniques improve inter-institutional agreement in interpretation of dobutamine stress echocardiograms. Eur Heart J 2002; 23:821–829.
5. Hoffmann R, Lethen H, Marwick T, et al. Standardized guidelines for the interpretation of dobutamine echocardiography reduce interinstitutional variance in interpretation. Am J Cardiol 1998; 82:1520–1524.
6. Arnese M, Fioretti PM, Cornel JH, et al. Akinesis becoming dyskinesis during high-dose dobutamine stress echocardiography: A marker of myocardial ischemia or a mechanical phenomenon? Am J Cardiol 1994; 73:896–899.
7. Attenhofer CH, Pellikka PA, Oh JK, et al. Comparison of ischemic response during exercise and dobutamine echocardiography in patients with left main coronary artery disease. J Am Coll Cardiol 1996; 27:1171–1177.
8. Bach DS, Muller DW, Gros BJ, et al. False positive dobutamine stress echocardiograms: Characterization of clinical, echocardiographic and angiographic findings. J Am Coll Cardiol 1994; 24:928–933.
9. Attenhofer CH, Pellikka PA, Oh JK, et al. Is review of videotape necessary after review of digitized cine-loop images in stress echocardiography? A prospective study in 306 patients. J Am Soc Echocardiogr 1997; 10:179–184.
10. Marwick TH, D'Hondt AM, Mairesse GH, et al. Comparative ability of dobutamine and exercise stress in inducing myocardial ischaemia in active patients. Br Heart J 1994; 72:31–38.
11. Rallidis L, Cokkinos P, Tousoulis D, et al. Comparison of dobutamine and treadmill exercise echocardiography in inducing ischemia in patients with coronary artery disease. J Am Coll Cardiol 1997; 30:1660–1668.
12. Fioretti PM, Poldermans D, Salustri A, et al. Atropine increases the accuracy of dobutamine stress echocardiography in patients taking beta-blockers. Eur Heart J 1994; 15:355–360.
13. Dagianti A, Penco M, Bandiera A, et al. Clinical application of exercise stress echocardiography: Supine bicycle or treadmill? Am J Cardiol 1998; 81:62G–67G.

14. Klein J, Cheo S, Berman DS, et al. Pathophysiologic factors governing the variability of ischemic responses to treadmill and bicycle exercise. Am Heart J 1994; 128:948–955.
15. Noguchi Y, Nagata-Kobayashi S, Stahl JE, et al. A meta-analytic comparison of echocardiographic stressors. Int J Cardiovasc Imaging 2005; 21:189–207.
16. Agati L, Arata L, Luongo R, et al. Assessment of severity of coronary narrowings by quantitative exercise echocardiography and comparison with quantitative arteriography. Am J Cardiol 1991; 67:1201–1207.
17. Beleslin BD, Ostojic M, Djordjevic-Dikic A, et al. Integrated evaluation of relation between coronary lesion features and stress echocardiography results: The importance of coronary lesion morphology. J Am Coll Cardiol 1999; 33:717–726.
18. Geleijnse ML, Elhendy A. Can stress echocardiography compete with perfusion scintigraphy in the detection of coronary artery disease and cardiac risk assessment? Eur J Echocardiogr 2000; 1:12–21.
19. Marwick TH, Nemec JJ, Stewart WJ, et al. Diagnosis of coronary artery disease using exercise echocardiography and positron emission tomography: Comparison and analysis of discrepant results. J Am Soc Echocardiogr 1992; 5:231–238.
20. Santoro GM, Sciagra R, Buonamici P, et al. Head-to-head comparison of exercise stress testing, pharmacologic stress echocardiography, and perfusion tomography as first-line examination for chest pain in patients without history of coronary artery disease. J Nucl Cardiol 1998; 5:19–27.
21. Baptista J, Arnese M, Roelandt JR, et al. Quantitative coronary angiography in the estimation of the functional significance of coronary stenosis: Correlations with dobutamine-atropine stress test. J Am Coll Cardiol 1994; 23:1434–1439.
22. Bartunek J, Marwick TH, Rodrigues AC, et al. Dobutamine-induced wall motion abnormalities: Correlations with myocardial fractional flow reserve and quantitative coronary angiography. J Am Coll Cardiol 1996; 27:1429–1436.
23. Picano E, Pingitore A, Conti U, et al. Enhanced sensitivity for detection of coronary artery disease by addition of atropine to dipyridamole echocardiography. Eur Heart J 1993; 14:1216–1222.
24. Danzi GB, Pirelli S, Mauri L, et al. Which variable of stenosis severity best describes the significance of an isolated left anterior descending coronary artery lesion? Correlation between quantitative coronary angiography, intracoronary Doppler measurements and high dose dipyridamole echocardiography. J Am Coll Cardiol 1998; 31:526–533.
25. Picano E, Severi S, Michelassi C, et al. Prognostic importance of dipyridamole-echocardiography test in coronary artery disease. Circulation 1989; 80:450–457.
26. Poldermans D, Arnese M, Fioretti PM, et al. Improved cardiac risk stratification in major vascular surgery with dobutamine-atropine stress echocardiography. J Am Coll Cardiol 1995; 26:648–653.
27. Senior R, Lahiri A. Enhanced detection of myocardial ischemia by stress dobutamine echocardiography utilizing the "biphasic" response of wall thickening during low and high dose dobutamine infusion. J Am Coll Cardiol 1995; 26:26–32.
28. Marwick TH. Stress echocardiography. In Topol E. Textbook of Cardiovascular Medicine, 3rd edition. Lippincott, Williams and Wilkins, Philadelphia 2007.
29. Armstrong WF, O'Donnell J, Dillon JC, et al. Complementary value of two-dimensional exercise echocardiography to routine treadmill exercise testing. Ann Intern Med 1986; 105:829–835.
30. Nesto RW, Kowalchuk GJ. The ischemic cascade: temporal sequence of hemodynamic, electrocardiographic and symptomatic expressions of ischemia. Am J Cardiol 1987; 59:23C–30C.
31. Sketch MH, Mohiuddin SM, Lynch JD, et al. Significant sex differences in the correlation of electrocardiographic exercise testing and coronary arteriograms. Am J Cardiol 1975; 36:169–173.
32. Marwick TH, Anderson T, Williams MJ, et al. Exercise echocardiography is an accurate and cost-efficient technique for detection of coronary artery disease in women. J Am Coll Cardiol 1995; 26:335–341.

33. Marwick TH, Torelli J, Harjai K, et al. Influence of left ventricular hypertrophy on detection of coronary artery disease using exercise echocardiography. J Am Coll Cardiol 1995; 26:1180–1186.

34. Fleischmann KE, Hunink MG, Kuntz KM, et al. Exercise echocardiography or exercise SPECT imaging? A meta-analysis of diagnostic test performance. JAMA 1998; 280:913–920.

35. Armstrong WF. Stress echocardiography for detection of coronary artery disease. Circulation 1991; 84:I43–I49.

36. Salustri A, Pozzoli MM, Hermans W, et al. Relationship between exercise echocardiography and perfusion single-photon emission computed tomography in patients with single-vessel coronary artery disease. Am Heart J 1992; 124:75–83.

37. Marwick T, Willemart B, D'Hondt AM, et al. Selection of the optimal nonexercise stress for the evaluation of ischemic regional myocardial dysfunction and malperfusion. Comparison of dobutamine and adenosine using echocardiography and 99mTc-MIBI single photon emission computed tomography. Circulation 1993; 87:345–354.

38. O'Keefe JH Jr., Barnhart CS, Bateman TM. Comparison of stress echocardiography and stress myocardial perfusion scintigraphy for diagnosing coronary artery disease and assessing its severity. Am J Cardiol 1995; 75:25D–34D.

39. Quinones MA, Verani MS, Haichin RM, et al. Exercise echocardiography versus 201Tl single-photon emission computed tomography in evaluation of coronary artery disease. Analysis of 292 patients. Circulation 1992; 85:1026–1031.

40. Kwok Y, Kim C, Grady D, et al. Meta-analysis of exercise testing to detect coronary artery disease in women. Am J Cardiol 1999; 83:660–666.

41. Fragasso G, Lu C, Dabrowski P, et al. Comparison of stress/rest myocardial perfusion tomography, dipyridamole and dobutamine stress echocardiography for the detection of coronary disease in hypertensive patients with chest pain and positive exercise test. J Am Coll Cardiol 1999; 34:441–447.

42. Klocke FJ, Baird MG, Bateman TM, et al. ACC/AHA/ASNC guidelines for the clinical use of cardiac radionuclide imaging: a report of the American College of Cardiology/American Heart Association Task Force on Practice Guidelines (ACC/AHA/ASNC Committee to Revise the 1995 Guidelines for the Clinical Use of Cardiac Radionuclide Imaging). (2003). American College of Cardiology Web Site. Available at: http://www.acc.org/clinical/guidelines/radio/rni_fulltext.pdf.

43. Biagini E, Shaw LJ, Poldermans D, et al. Accuracy of non-invasive techniques for diagnosis of coronary artery disease and prediction of cardiac events in patients with left bundle branch block: A meta-analysis. Eur J Nucl Med Mol Imaging 2006; 33:1442–1451.

44. Pasquet A, Armstrong G, Rimmerman C, et al. Correlation of myocardial Doppler velocity response to exercise with independent evidence of myocardial ischemia by dual-isotope single-photon emission computed tomography. Am J Cardiol 2000; 85:536–542.

45. Cain P, Baglin T, Case C, et al. Application of tissue Doppler to interpretation of dobutamine echocardiography and comparison with quantitative coronary angiography. Am J Cardiol 2001; 87:525–531.

46. Voigt JU, Exner B, Schmiedehausen K, et al. Strain-rate imaging during dobutamine stress echocardiography provides objective evidence of inducible ischemia. Circulation 2003; 107:2120–2126.

47. Voigt JU, Nixdorff U, Bogdan R, et al. Comparison of deformation imaging and velocity imaging for detecting regional inducible ischaemia during dobutamine stress echocardiography. Eur Heart J 2004; 25:1517–1525.

48. Ingul CB, Stoylen A, Slordahl SA, et al. Automated analysis of myocardial deformation at dobutamine stress echocardiography: An angiographic validation. J Am Coll Cardiol 2007; 49:1651–1659.

49. Bjork Ingul C, Rozis E, Slordahl SA, et al. Incremental value of strain rate imaging to wall motion analysis for prediction of outcome in patients undergoing dobutamine stress echocardiography. Circulation 2007; 115:1252–1259.

50. Hanekom L, Cho GY, Leano R, et al. Comparison of two-dimensional speckle and tissue Doppler strain measurement during dobutamine stress echocardiography: An angiographic correlation. Eur Heart J 2007;28:1765–72.

51. Porter TR, Xie F, Kricsfeld A, et al. Improved endocardial border resolution during dobutamine stress echocardiography with intravenous sonicated dextrose albumin. J Am Coll Cardiol 1994; 23:1440–1443.

52. Shaw LJ, Monaghan MJ, Nihoyannopolous P. Clinical and economic outcomes assessment with myocardial contrast echocardiography. Heart 1999; 82(suppl 3): III16–III21.

53. Ten Cate FJ. Usefulness of ultrasound contrast for image enhancement during stress echocardiography. Echocardiography 2002; 19:621–625.

54. Rainbird AJ, Mulvagh SL, Oh JK, et al. Contrast dobutamine stress echocardiography: Clinical practice assessment in 300 consecutive patients. J Am Soc Echocardiogr 2001; 14:378–385.

55. Falcone RA, Marcovitz PA, Perez JE, et al. Intravenous albunex during dobutamine stress echocardiography: Enhanced localization of left ventricular endocardial borders. Am Heart J 1995; 130:254–258.

56. Schroder K, Agrawal R, Voller H, et al. Improvement of endocardial border delineation in suboptimal stress-echocardiograms using the new left heart contrast agent SH U 508 A. Int J Card Imaging 1994; 10:45–51.

57. Dolan MS, Riad K, El-Shafei A, et al. Effect of intravenous contrast for left ventricular opacification and border definition on sensitivity and specificity of dobutamine stress echocardiography compared with coronary angiography in technically difficult patients. Am Heart J 2001; 142:908–915.

58. Kaul S, Senior R, Dittrich H, et al. Detection of coronary artery disease with myocardial contrast echocardiography: Comparison with 99mTc-sestamibi single-photon emission computed tomography. Circulation 1997; 96:785–792.

59. Dijkmans PA, Senior R, Becher H, et al. Myocardial contrast echocardiography evolving as a clinically feasible technique for accurate, rapid, and safe assessment of myocardial perfusion: the evidence so far. J Am Coll Cardiol 2006; 48: 2168–2177.

60. Moir S, Haluska BA, Jenkins C, et al. Incremental benefit of myocardial contrast to combined dipyridamole-exercise stress echocardiography for the assessment of coronary artery disease. Circulation 2004; 110:1108–1113.

61. Marwick TH. Stress echocardiography with non-exercise techniques: Principles, protocols, interpretation and clinical applications. In Otto CM. The Practice of Clinical Echocardiography 3rd ed. Saunders Elsevier, Philadelphia 2007.

62. San Roman JA, Vilacosta I, Castillo JA, et al. Dipyridamole and dobutamine-atropine stress echocardiography in the diagnosis of coronary artery disease. Comparison with exercise stress test, analysis of agreement, and impact of antianginal treatment. Chest 1996; 110:1248–1254.

63. Kisacik HL, Ozdemir K, Altinyay E, et al. Comparison of exercise stress testing with simultaneous dobutamine stress echocardiography and technetium-99m isonitrile single-photon emission computerized tomography for diagnosis of coronary artery disease. Eur Heart J 1996; 17:113–119.

64. Pozzoli MM, Fioretti PM, Salustri A, et al. Exercise echocardiography and technetium-99m MIBI single-photon emission computed tomography in the detection of coronary artery disease. Am J Cardiol 1991; 67:350–355.

65. Galanti G, Sciagra R, Comeglio M, et al. Diagnostic accuracy of peak exercise echocardiography in coronary artery disease: Comparison with thallium-201 myocardial scintigraphy. Am Heart J 1991; 122:1609–1616.

66. Hecht HS, DeBord L, Shaw R, et al. Supine bicycle stress echocardiography versus tomographic thallium-201 exercise imaging for the detection of coronary artery disease. J Am Soc Echocardiogr 1993; 6:177–185.

67. Takeuchi M, Araki M, Nakashima Y, et al. Comparison of dobutamine stress echocardiography and stress thallium-201 single-photon emission computed tomography for detecting coronary artery disease. J Am Soc Echocardiogr 1993; 6:593–602.

68. San Roman JA, Rollan MJ, Vilacosta I, et al. Echocardiography and MIBI-SPECT scintigraphy during dobutamine infusion in the diagnosis of coronary disease. Rev Esp Cardiol 1995; 48:606–614.

69. Parodi G, Picano E, Marcassa C, et al. High dose dipyridamole myocardial imaging: Simultaneous sestamibi scintigraphy and two-dimensional echocardiography in the detection and evaluation of coronary artery disease. Italian Group of Nuclear Cardiology. Coron Artery Dis 1999; 10:177–184.

70. Smart SC, Bhatia A, Hellman R, et al. Dobutamine-atropine stress echocardiography and dipyridamole sestamibi scintigraphy for the detection of coronary artery disease: Limitations and concordance. J Am Coll Cardiol 2000; 36:1265–1273.

71. Sawada SG, Segar DS, Ryan T, et al. Echocardiographic detection of coronary artery disease during dobutamine infusion. Circulation 1991; 83:1605–1614.

72. Marcovitz PA, Armstrong WF. Accuracy of dobutamine stress echocardiography in detecting coronary artery disease. Am J Cardiol 1992; 69:1269–1273.

73. Marwick T, D'Hondt AM, Baudhuin T, et al. Optimal use of dobutamine stress for the detection and evaluation of coronary artery disease: combination with echocardiography or scintigraphy, or both? J Am Coll Cardiol 1993; 22:159–167.

74. Takeuchi M, Araki M, Nakashima Y, Kuroiwa A. Comparison of dobutamine stress echocardiography and stress thallium-201 single-photon emission computed tomography for detecting coronary artery disease. J Am Soc Echocardiogr 1993; 6:593–602.

75. Beleslin BD, Ostojic M, Stepanovic J, et al. Stress echocardiography in the detection of myocardial ischemia. Head-to-head comparison of exercise, dobutamine, and dipyridamole tests. Circulation 1994; 90:1168–1176.

76. Ostojic M, Picano E, Beleslin B, et al. Dipyridamole-dobutamine echocardiography: a novel test for the detection of milder forms of coronary artery disease. J Am Coll Cardiol 1994; 23:1115–1122.

77. Pingitore A, Picano E, Colosso MQ, et al. The atropine factor in pharmacologic stress echocardiography. Echo Persantine (EPIC) and Echo Dobutamine International Cooperative (EDIC) Study Groups. J Am Coll Cardiol 1996; 27:1164–1170.

78. Ling LH, Pellikka PA, Mahoney DW, et al. Atropine augmentation in dobutamine stress echocardiography: role and incremental value in a clinical practice setting. J Am Coll Cardiol 1996; 28:551–557.

79. San Roman JA, Vilacosta I, Castillo JA, et al. Dipyridamole and dobutamine-atropine stress echocardiography in the diagnosis of coronary artery disease. Comparison with exercise stress test, analysis of agreement, and impact of antianginal treatment. Chest 1996; 110:1248–1254.

80. Anthopoulos LP, Bonou MS, Sioras EP, Kranidis AI, Kardaras FG, Antonellis IP. Echocardiographic detection of the extent of coronary artery disease in the elderly using dobutamine and adenosine infusion. Coron Artery Dis 1997; 8:633–643.

81. Dionisopoulos PN, Collins JD, Smart SC, Knickelbine TA, Sagar KB. The value of dobutamine stress echocardiography for the detection of coronary artery disease in women. J Am Soc Echocardiogr 1997; 10:811–817.

82. Elhendy A, Geleijnse ML, van Domburg RT, et al. Gender differences in the accuracy of dobutamine stress echocardiography for the diagnosis of coronary artery disease. Am J Cardiol 1997; 80:1414–1418.

83. Hennessy TG, Codd MB, McCarthy C, Kane G, McCann HA, Sugrue DD. Dobutamine stress echocardiography in the detection of coronary artery disease in a clinical practice setting. Int J Cardiol 1997; 62:55–62.

84. Nagel E, Lehmkuhl HB, Bocksch W, et al. Noninvasive diagnosis of ischemia-induced wall motion abnormalities with the use of high-dose dobutamine stress MRI: comparison with dobutamine stress echocardiography. Circulation 1999; 99:763–770.

85. Beleslin BD, Ostojic M, Djordjevic-Dikic A, et al. Integrated evaluation of relation between coronary lesion features and stress echocardiography results: the importance of coronary lesion morphology. J Am Coll Cardiol 1999; 33:717–726.

86. Picano E, Severi S, Lattanzi F, et al. [The diagnostic and prognostic value of echo-dipyridamole in patients with suspected coronary disease: a comparison with the stress test]. G Ital Cardiol 1991; 21:621–632.

87. Severi S, Picano E, Michelassi C, et al. Diagnostic and prognostic value of dipyridamole echocardiography in patients with suspected coronary artery disease. Comparison with exercise electrocardiography. Circulation 1994; 89:1160–1173.

88. Picano E, Pingitore A, Conti U, et al. Enhanced sensitivity for detection of coronary artery disease by addition of atropine to dipyridamole echocardiography. Eur Heart J 1993; 14:1216–1222.

89. Picano E, Lattanzi F, Masini M, Distante A, L'Abbate A. Comparison of the high-dose dipyridamole-echocardiography test and exercise two-dimensional echocardiography for diagnosis of coronary artery disease. Am J Cardiol 1987; 59:539–542.

90. Hoffmann R, Lethen H, Kleinhans E, Weiss M, Flachskampf FA, Hanrath P. Comparative evaluation of bicycle and dobutamine stress echocardiography with perfusion scintigraphy and bicycle electrocardiogram for identification of coronary artery disease. Am J Cardiol 1993; 72:555–559.

91. Cohen JL, Ottenweller JE, George AK, Duvvuri S. Comparison of dobutamine and exercise echocardiography for detecting coronary artery disease. Am J Cardiol 1993; 72:1226–1231.

92. Marangelli V, Iliceto S, Piccinni G, De Martino G, Sorgente L, Rizzon P. Detection of coronary artery disease by digital stress echocardiography: comparison of exercise, transesophageal atrial pacing and dipyridamole echocardiography. J Am Coll Cardiol 1994; 24:117–124.

93. Marwick TH, D'Hondt AM, Mairesse GH, et al. Comparative ability of dobutamine and exercise stress in inducing myocardial ischaemia in active patients. Br Heart J 1994; 72:31–38.

94. Dagianti A, Penco M, Agati L, et al. Stress echocardiography: comparison of exercise, dipyridamole and dobutamine in detecting and predicting the extent of coronary artery disease. J Am Coll Cardiol 1995; 26:18–25.

95. Kisacik HL, Ozdemir K, Altinyay E, et al. Comparison of exercise stress testing with simultaneous dobutamine stress echocardiography and technetium-99m isonitrile single-photon emission computerized tomography for diagnosis of coronary artery disease. Eur Heart J 1996; 17:113–119.

96. Rallidis L, Cokkinos P, Tousoulis D, Nihoyannopoulos P. Comparison of dobutamine and treadmill exercise echocardiography in inducing ischemia in patients with coronary artery disease. J Am Coll Cardiol 1997; 30:1660–1668.

97. Santoro GM, Sciagra R, Buonamici P, et al. Head-to-head comparison of exercise stress testing, pharmacologic stress echocardiography, and perfusion tomography as first-line examination for chest pain in patients without history of coronary artery disease. J Nucl Cardiol 1998; 5:19–27.

98. Marwick T, Willemart B, D'Hondt AM, et al. Selection of the optimal nonexercise stress for the evaluation of ischemic regional myocardial dysfunction and malperfusion. Comparison of dobutamine and adenosine using echocardiography and 99mTc-MIBI single photon emission computed tomography. Circulation 1993; 87: 345–354.

99. Previtali M, Lanzarini L, Fetiveau R, et al. Comparison of dobutamine stress echocardiography, dipyridamole stress echocardiography and exercise stress testing for diagnosis of coronary artery disease. Am J Cardiol 1993; 72:865–870.

100. Loimaala A, Groundstroem K, Pasanen M, Oja P, Vuori I. Comparison of bicycle, heavy isometric, dipyridamole-atropine and dobutamine stress echocardiography for diagnosis of myocardial ischemia. Am J Cardiol 1999; 84:1396–1400.

101. Fragasso G, Lu C, Dabrowski P, Pagnotta P, Sheiban I, Chierchia SL. Comparison of stress/rest myocardial perfusion tomography, dipyridamole and dobutamine stress echocardiography for the detection of coronary disease in hypertensive patients with chest pain and positive exercise test. J Am Coll Cardiol 1999; 34:441–447.

102. Pozzoli MM, Fioretti PM, Salustri A, Reijs AE, Roelandt JR. Exercise echocardiography and technetium-99m MIBI single-photon emission computed tomography in the detection of coronary artery disease. Am J Cardiol 1991; 67:350–355.

103. Galanti G, Sciagra R, Comeglio M, et al. Diagnostic accuracy of peak exercise echocardiography in coronary artery disease: comparison with thallium-201 myocardial scintigraphy. Am Heart J 1991; 122:1609–1616.

104. Quinones MA, Verani MS, Haichin RM, Mahmarian JJ, Suarez J, Zoghbi WA. Exercise echocardiography versus 201Tl single-photon emission computed tomography in evaluation of coronary artery disease. Analysis of 292 patients. Circulation 1992; 85:1026–1031.

105. Hecht HS, DeBord L, Shaw R, et al. Supine bicycle stress echocardiography versus tomographic thallium-201 exercise imaging for the detection of coronary artery disease. J Am Soc Echocardiogr 1993; 6:177–185.

106. Senior R, Sridhara BS, Anagnostou E, Handler C, Raftery EB, Lahiri A. Synergistic value of simultaneous stress dobutamine sestamibi single-photon-emission computerized tomography and echocardiography in the detection of coronary artery disease. Am Heart J 1994; 128:713–718.

107. Ho FM, Huang PJ, Liau CS, et al. Dobutamine stress echocardiography compared with dipyridamole thallium-201 single-photon emission computed tomography in detecting coronary artery disease. Eur Heart J 1995; 16:570–575.

108. San Roman JA, Rollan MJ, Vilacosta I, et al. [Echocardiography and MIBI-SPECT scintigraphy during dobutamine infusion in the diagnosis of coronary disease]. Rev Esp Cardiol 1995; 48:606–614.

109. Huang PJ, Ho YL, Wu CC, et al. Simultaneous dobutamine stress echocardiography and thallium-201 perfusion imaging for the detection of coronary artery disease. Cardiology 1997; 88:556–562.

110. Parodi G, Picano E, Marcassa C, et al. High dose dipyridamole myocardial imaging: simultaneous sestamibi scintigraphy and two-dimensional echocardiography in the detection and evaluation of coronary artery disease. Italian Group of Nuclear Cardiology. Coron Artery Dis 1999; 10:177–184.

111. Smart SC, Bhatia A, Hellman R, et al. Dobutamine-atropine stress echocardiography and dipyridamole sestamibi scintigraphy for the detection of coronary artery disease: limitations and concordance. J Am Coll Cardiol 2000; 36:1265–1273.

7 Detection of Myocardial Viability

Paolo Colonna

Institute of Cardiology, Policlinico Hospital, Bari, Italy

I. THE POSTINFARCTION VIABLE MYOCARDIUM

In the course of acute myocardial infarction (AMI), the presence of regional contractile dysfunction of the left ventricle is not always an index of myocardial necrosis. In fact the finding of a dyssynergic area of myocardium can also indicate an area of "dysfunctioning, but still viable" myocardium. The definition of "viable myocardium" is applied to two different pathophysiologic conditions:

(a) the "stunned myocardium" that characterizes a postischemic dysfunctional myocardium in the presence of normal regional blood flow (Fig. 1A) (1);

(b) the "hibernating myocardium", characterized by reversible loss of contractility in the presence of reduced blood flow in comparison to normal regional values (Fig. 1B); in this condition, the myocardium reacts with downregulation of the contractile activity to the reduction of flow to reduce the myocardial oxygen consumption at most ("smart heart") (2).

Often these two conditions coexist in postinfarction reperfusion: after spontaneous coronary recanalization, after pharmacologic thrombolysis, or after primary angioplasty. However, between these two conditions there are some clinical and physiological differences simplified in the attached table (Fig. 2).

The AMI determines an alteration of the regional contractile function that can be reversible or not, in relation to (*i*) the presence of collaterals at the moment of coronary occlusion (3); (*ii*) the rapidity with which reperfusion is obtained; (*iii*) the integrity of the microcirculation (4); and (*iv*) the amount of coronary flow after reperfusion (Fig. 3).

In the age of thrombolysis or primary angioplasty, there is a high probability that the myocardial damage is reversible, thanks to the early reperfusion. The recent improvement in different diagnostic techniques allowed the development of a model for a "temporal cascade after coronary occlusion" including anatomic and functional damages of microvasculature and myocytes (Fig. 4). Therefore, the extent of echocardiographic myocardial dysfunction estimated in the early postinfarction phase does not always correspond to the real histological myocardial damage; in fact, the performance of sequential echocardiograms after thrombolytic therapy showed that myocardial segments with reversible dysfunction recover after days, until 4 weeks.

The importance of studying the postischemic myocardial viability is evident since 1985, when Rahimtoola firstly described the hibernating myocardium like a dysfunctional myocardium due to chronic ischemia that reverts after reflow in minutes or days (2). It is well known that the prognosis of patients with AMI is closely tied to the left ventricular systolic function and that in chronic ischemic myocardial dysfunction, such prognosis is altered by the presence

Myocardial stunning

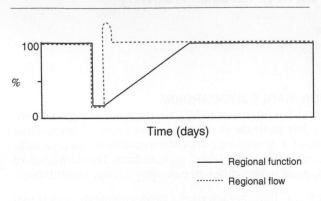

——— Regional function
········ Regional flow

Myocardial hibernation

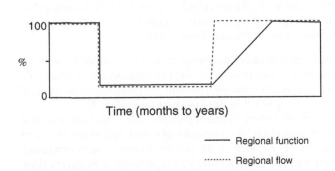

——— Regional function
········ Regional flow

FIGURE 1 Schematic of myocardial blood flow and regional function in the two different pathophysiologic conditions of viable myocardium. In the "stunned myocardium" (top graph), there is a postischemic depression of regional myocardial function in the presence of normal regional blood flow; in the "hibernating myocardium" (bottom graph), there is a prolonged reduction of regional myocardial function in the presence of reduced regional blood flow.

of viable myocardium (5). Therefore, the early and precise identification of a reversible left ventricular dysfunction appears much useful for the prognosis and therapeutic approach of ischemic patients.

II. HOW TO STUDY MYOCARDIAL VIABILITY

The diagnostic tests most commonly used for the assessment of the viable myocardium in clinical practice are as follows:

- Echocardiography during infusion of dobutamine
- Computed tomography with emission of single photon (thallium or technetium—SPECT)
- Positron emission tomography (PET)

	Stunning	**Hibernation**
Myocardial contractile function	Reduced at rest. Improvement with dobutamine	Reduced at rest (downregulation). Improvement (often "biphasic response") with dobutamine
Contractility at follow up	Full spontaneous recovery	Mostly recovery with revascularization
Time of contratile recovery	Hours to days; merges with delayed recovery from ischemia over weeks	After revascularization: days to hours to months
Coronary blood flow	Normal (postischemic); variable coronary flow reserve	Reduced; impaired coronary flow reserve
Myocardial metabolism and calcium	Fatty acid metabolism + cytosolic calcium overload (contractile proteins damage)	Reduced metabolism ("smart heart"); complex defects in calcium cycling (vb Heusch)

FIGURE 2 Table indicating pathophysiologic aspects of contractility, vascularization, and metabolism of the two different conditions of viable myocardium.

- Magnetic resonance imaging with wall motion analysis (during infusion of dobutamine) and/or myocardial perfusion analysis after gadolinium infusion.
- Myocardial contrast echocardiography

Concerning the dobutamine echocardiography (here analyzed in detail because of the theme of this textbook), the infusion of catecholamine is able to improve wall thickening in postischemic dysfunctional but viable myocardium, thus allowing the differentiation of viable myocardium from the necrosis (6). Hence the rationale to employ low-dose dobutamine in the presence of viable myocardium is (a) after myocardial infarction (stunned myocardium) and (b) in patients with chronic coronary disease (hibernating myocardium).

Factors influencing presence / extension of viable myocardium

- Time to reperfusion
- Collateral circulation
- Microvascular integrity
- Entity of blood flow after reperfusion (eventual damage from abrupt recanalization)

FIGURE 3 Clinical factors influencing the presence and extension of viable myocardium.

Temporal cascade after coronary occlusion

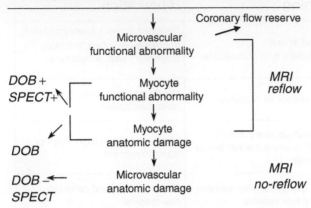

FIGURE 4 Hypothetical model for a "temporal cascade after coronary occlusion" including anatomic and functional damage of microvasculature and myocytes, illustrating the usefulness of different cardiac imaging techniques.

The echodobutamine has the advantage of being a simple procedure, highly specific, with great spatial resolution, widely available, safe, and inexpensive compared to the scintigraphic techniques, especially the positron emission tomography (PET), which has been considered the gold standard in the study of the viable myocardium. Moreover it is capable of assessing viability at low doses and ischemia at higher doses and it is predictive of clinical outcomes (Fig. 5).

Conversely, as the uptake of thallium-201 and technetium-99 m from myocytes is an active process and depends on regional flow and myocytes membrane integrity, myocardial scintigraphy also allows distinguishing the viable myocardium from the scar with great precision. Several techniques such as early (3–4 hours) or late (8–72 hours) redistribution of thallium after stress or thallium reinjection after the early study are used. The late redistribution of thallium (without reinjection) is an accurate index of viable myocardium, even if it tends to overestimate the entity of the myocardial necrosis; therefore, the method of the reinjection appears more accurate in characterizing residual myocardial viability.

However, the straight method for the demonstration of viable myocardium is the one based on the use of PET. This technique allows an accurate evaluation of the regional distribution of tracing of flow and metabolism. The viable myocardium is identified in two phases: in the first, regional myocardial flow is quantified with tracing of flow (N 13-ammonia, rubidium-82, marked water with O15) and in the second phase, the metabolic activity is indirectly determined through the uptake of 18F-fluorodeoxyglucose (18F-FDG). The normal FDG uptake in regions with reduced flow (flow/metabolism mismatch) identifies the hibernating myocardium.

Several authors compared sensitivity, specificity, and predictive value of all the available techniques in the postischemic myocardial dysfunction (hibernating myocardium). The result of a meta-analysis of the above techniques for the prediction of functional recovery after revascularization is supplied in Figure 6 (7).

Technique	Advantages	Limitations
SPECT imaging	High sensitivity for predicting improved function after revascularization Uses quantitative objective criteria Predictive of clinical outcomes in a large number of studies	Reduced spatial resolution and sensitivity in comparison to PET Areas of attenuation (e.g., inferior wall on "Tc-sestamibi scans) misconstrued as nonviability Cannot separate endocardial from epicardial viability Lower specificity than dobutamine echocardiography for predicting improved function after revascularization
PET imaging	Simultaneous assessment of perfusion and metabolism Highly sensitive and specific No attenuation problems Absolute blood flow can be measured Predictive of outcomes	Lower speciflcity than dobutamine echocardiography Cannot separate endocardial from epicardial viability High cost and highly sophisticated technology Limited availability
Dobutamine echocardiography	Higher specificity than nuclear techniques Viability assessed at low doses and ischemia at higher doses Evaluation of mitral regurgitation Good spatial resolution Predictive of clinical outcomes Widely available with lower cost	Poor windows in small percent of patients Lower sensitivity than nuclear techniques Viable regions with absent flow reserve will not show increased thickening during dobutamine stimulation Reliance on visual assessment of wall thickening
Myocardial contrast echocardiography	Microcirculatory integrity evaluated as well as systolic thickening Better estimation of extent of viability than functional assessment alone Precise delineation of area of necrosis Viability assessed in the presence of total coronary occlusion	Difficult windows in 30% of patients Attenuation problems Scant clinical data available

FIGURE 5 Table indicating advantages and limitations of different imaging techniques in detecting myocardial viability.

III. LOW-DOSE DOBUTAMINE ECHOCARDIOGRAPHY: HOW TO PERFORM THE PROTOCOL

The dobutamine echocardiography test utilizes the response of the cardiac muscle to the β-receptor stimulus, obtained with the intravenous infusion of

Table Sensitivity and Specificity for the Different Imaging Techniques (Based on Weighted Mean Values from Available Studies)

	No. of pts	Sensitivity (%)	95% CI	99% CI	Specificity (%)	95% CI	99% CI
Tc-99m MIBI	207	83	78–87	77–89	69	63–74	61–76
LDDE	448	84	82–86	81–87	81	79–84	79–84
T1-201 reinjection	209	86	83–89	82–90	47	43–51	42–52
F-18 FDG PET	332	88	84–91	83–92	73	69–77	69–77
Tl-201 rest–redistribution	145	90	87–93	86–94	54	49–60	48–61

CI, condifence interval; F-18 FDG, fluorine-18 fluorodeoxyglucose; LDDE, low-dose dobutamine echocardiography; Tc-99m MIBI, technetium-99m sestamibi; T1-201, thallium-201.

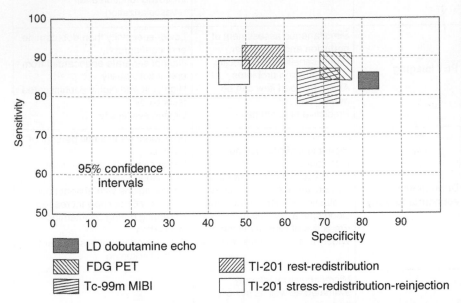

FIGURE 6 Table and graph indicating sensitivity and specificity of different imaging techniques for the prediction of functional recovery after revascularization in the hibernating myocardium. *Source*: Adapted from Ref. 7.

dobutamine. Among the effects of sympatomymetic amines on sympatic receptors, the dobutamine has a selective effect on β1-receptors (Fig. 7).

Thanks to the positive inotropic and chronotropic effects of this drug, the myocardium is at first stimulated to an energetic contraction (low dose, until 15 μg/kg/min) for the prevailing inotropic effect, with a modest increase in arterial systolic pressure. Later on, for the continued β-stimulation, the chronotropic positive effect occurs (high dose, until 40 μg/kg/min), with consequent increase of double product and oxygen consumption, obtaining the ischemic action of the test (Fig. 8).

The dobutamine echocardiography test has a precise intravenous infusion protocol, very well standardized after the early studies (6). The low-dose

Effects of sympatomymetic amines on sympatic receptors

	α	β1	β2
Isoproterenol	0	+++	+++
Adrenalin	++	+++	++
Dopamine	+++	+++	0
Dobutamine	+	+++	+

FIGURE 7 Effects of sympatomymetic amines on sympatic receptors.

echodobutamine protocol is performed with the intravenous administration through an infusion pump of increasing doses of dobutamine, starting at 5 μg/kg/min, which is doubled to 10 μg/kg/min after 5 minutes (Fig. 9). If the twofold information is required (myocardial viability at low dose and myocardial ischemia at high dose), the protocol goes on with the standard high-dose echodobutamine, with increases of 10 μg/kg/min every 3 minutes until 40 μg/kg/min plus, 0.25 mg of atropine repeated every minute 4 times (Fig. 9).

Sequence of arterial systolic pressure (ASP) and heart rate (Hr) during dobutamine infusion

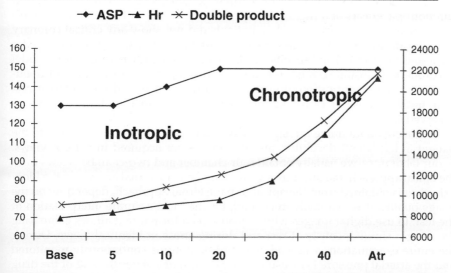

FIGURE 8 Changes in arterial systolic pressure and heart rate during dobutamine infusion for a protocol at low and high dosage.

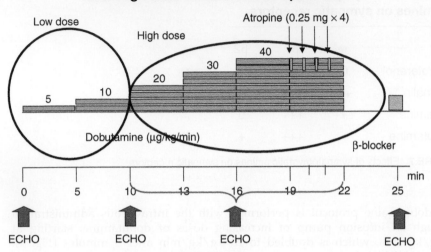

FIGURE 9 Schematic illustrating the infusion protocol and the time for echocardiography in the "low and high dosage dobutamine/atropine protocol."

Several studies searching the optimal dose of dobutamine for viable myocardium showed that the sensibility of the echodobutamine is higher with small dosages (e.g., 4 μg/kg/min) (8), while it is reduced with increasing dosages. A possible explanation for this lack of sensibility is due to myocardial ischemia generated by the high myocardial oxygen consumption (inotropic and chronotropic effects of a higher dosage of dobutamine) in the presence of critical coronary stenosis. In fact, when patients did not show any critical coronary stenosis, an intermediate–high dose of dobutamine (10 μg/kg/min) showed a great sensibility (83%) and specificity (86%) for viability (9). In dogs with a model of coronary occlusion (2–6 hours) and reperfusion, the necessary dose of dobutamine for the identification of viable myocardium increased with a larger risk area, until the dose of 15 μg/kg/min, when the maximal inotropic effect was observed (10).

During dobutamine infusion, the echocardiography is performed with the patient in left lateral decubitus, and the images are acquired in various views. In our laboratory, we usually obtain four-chamber and two-chamber views from the apical approach and short-axis view from the parasternal approach; the long-axis view is obtained from the apical or parasternal approach, depending on the image quality. It is extremely important, for the most accurate interpretation of the test, to use digital images with a quad screen format that allows comparing the images simultaneously at rest and during stress in identical views. During the entire examination, a 12-lead echocardiography is continuously monitored and the arterial pressure is measured every 3 minutes. After the end of the drug infusion, the patient is monitored for another 10–15 minutes, as dobutamine has a half-life of approximately 2 minutes and is completely metabolized or eliminated in 10–12 minutes.

At low dose, the classical end-points of the echodobutamine test are not achieved (see later), and the adverse effects do very rarely occur, although they are possible when infusing dobutamine at high dose.

IV. LOW-DOSE DOBUTAMINE ECHOCARDIOGRAPHY: HOW TO EVALUATE THE RESULTS

During the entire dobutamine echocardiography test, the regional myocardial wall motion and the contractile response are carefully estimated through qualitative and semiquantitative analysis of regional parietal systolic thickening according to the guidelines of the American Society of Echocardiography.

The dysfunctioning myocardium, identified as the portion of left ventricular wall akinetic, dyskinetic, or hypokinetic at rest, modifies in dose-dependent manner in response to dobutamine. The time–course response to dobutamine can be variable also in the presence of viability, depending on (a) the lumen patency of the coronary artery, (b) the extent of myocardial territory supplied by the responsible coronary, and (c) the eventual flow from collateral circulation.

Criteria for a positive viability response (namely, the presence of contractile reserve and viability) are:

(1) improvement of the wall motion in at least two contiguous segments;
(2) 20% reduction of the wall motion score index.

According to these criteria, the contractile reserve is present if the patient shows substantial improvement of regional parietal thickening to any dose of dobutamine, even if subsequently there is deterioration of function, caused by the occurrence of ischemia.

At least three patterns of myocardial response to dobutamine, useful to define the state of myocardial viability, have been characterized (loops 44–49):

- Monophasic positive response: progressive wall motion improvement at low and high doses, interpretable as the presence of myocardial viability combined to (a) an infarct-related coronary without significant residual stenosis or (b) with collateral flow adequate to guarantee wall motion improvement;
- Biphasic positive response: a contractile improvement at low dose and a deterioration at high dose; this is interpretable as the presence of myocardial viability (contractile reserve at low dose), combined to an infarct-related coronary with significant residual stenosis or inadequate regional collateral flow (viable myocardium at risk);
- Negative response: (absence of improvement during infusion of dobutamine), interpretable as not viable myocardium, area of potentially irreversible damage, or scarred myocardial infarction.

All the above patterns are often mixed with those obtained during the high-dose dobutamine echocardiography for the detection of ischemia, described in the appropriate chapter (Fig. 10) (11).

Indeed, the dose/response curve can vary continuously in the same area of myocardium, because it depends not only on the myocardial viability but also on other determining factors of contractility such as preload, afterload, heart

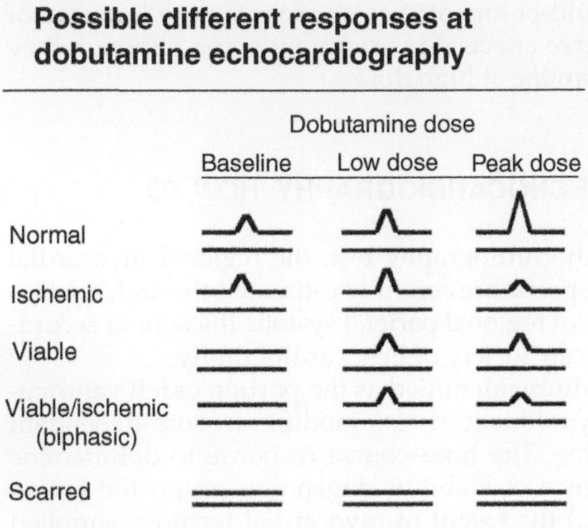

Possible different responses at
dobutamine echocardiography

	Dobutamine dose		
	Baseline	Low dose	Peak dose
Normal			
Ischemic			
Viable			
Viable/ischemic (biphasic)			
Scarred			

FIGURE 10 Schematic of the different responses at dobutamine echocardiography, obtained during the low- and high-dose protocol for the detection of myocardial viability and ischemia. The schematic illustrates a simplification of parasternal M-mode tracings. *Source*: Adapted from Ref. 11.

rate, and transmural extension of myocytes necrosis and viability (12). All these reasons can explain the possible occurrence of false-positive and false-negative responses at dobutamine echocardiography.

V. CLINICAL SIGNIFICANCE OF THE ECHODOBUTAMINE TEST
The clinical importance of the dobutamine echocardiography and of the other tests to evaluate myocardial viability relies on the interest to characterize at best patients with acute and chronic coronary artery disease and on the opportunity to obtain a functional myocardial recovery with medical therapy or revascularization.

Several studies have demonstrated the validity of dobutamine echocardiography in characterizing the stunned or hibernating myocardium in patients with acute and chronic left ventricular dysfunction. Furthermore, the high positive and negative predictive values of echodobutamine and of other viability tests in determining the recovery of the left-ventricle regional function over time and after myocardial revascularization (PTCA or CABG), have been pointed out (7,13). In fact, an early revascularization intervention has been shown to be very effective in patients showing myocardial viability (14). Moreover, benefits in quality of life and reduced heart failure symptoms for patients with myocardial viability after revascularization have also been demonstrated (15).

Besides the identification of viable myocardium, the quantification of reversible dysfunction is of great clinical importance; those patients with large amount of viable myocardium (more than six segments recovering during dobutamine echocardiography) have greater postrevascularization improvement in left ventricular systolic function and better prognosis as compared with those a small amount or without viable myocardium (16).

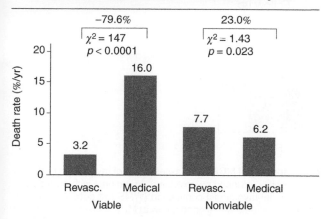

Myocardial viability testing and impact of revascularization on prognosis in patients with CAD and LV dysfunction: a meta-analysis

FIGURE 11 Graphs from a meta-analysis indicating the prognostic value of viability testing in order to aid clinical decision making (revascularization on prognosis in patients with CAD and LV dysfunction). *Source*: Adapted from Ref. 5.

Concerning the improvement of survival in patients revascularized with viable myocardium, a recent meta-analysis pooled 24 single-center studies examining the prognostic value of viability testing in order to aid clinical decision making in 3088 patients with severe coronary artery disease (CAD) and associated left ventricular dysfunction (mean ejection fraction 32 ± 8%) (5). It noted that in patients with myocardial viability, revascularization was associated with 79.6% reduction in annual mortality (16% vs. 3.2%, $p < 0.0001$) compared with medical treatment. In patients without viability, the mortality was intermediate, trending to higher rates with revascularization versus medical therapy (7.7% vs. 6.2%, p = NS). Patients with viability showed a direct relationship between severity of left ventricular dysfunction and magnitude of benefit with revascularization ($p < 0.001$) (Fig. 11).

Moreover, there was no measurable performance difference for predicting revascularization benefit between thallium perfusion imaging, 18F-FDG PET metabolic imaging and dobutamine echocardiography.

All these data show a strong association between myocardial viability on noninvasive testing and improved survival after revascularization and, therefore, strongly indicate the performance of dobutamine echo or other noninvasive tests for the best treatment of patients with chronic CAD and left ventricular dysfunction.

VI. THE MYOCARDIAL CONTRAST ECHOCARDIOGRAPHY TO STUDY MYOCARDIAL VIABILITY

In the end, it is interesting to describe a recently new echocardiographic technology, the myocardial contrast echocardiography (MCE), which is assuming an important role in the evaluation of the viable myocardium.

WMSi in the disfunctioning LV infarct area
(baseline, Dobut, Follow up)

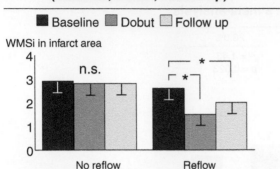

FIGURE 12   Graphs indicating the capability of MCE in the assessment of myocardial perfusion and in the prediction of myocardial viability (stunned myocardium). In patients with no reflow at MCE, there is no improvement in regional myocardial contraction (WMSI) at dobutamine echo and at follow up (absence of viability); in patients with a good reflow at MCE there is improvement both at dobutamine echo and at follow up (presence of viability). *Source*: Adapted from Ref. 17.

Different from the other techniques, the MCE allows estimating the anatomical and perfusional integrity of coronary microcirculation—a precise delineation of area of necrosis—even in the presence of total coronary occlusion (Fig. 5). Conversely this technique is limited by the inadequate echocardiographic windows in a substantial percentage of patients by some echocardiographic attenuation problems, and it is still missing sufficient clinical evidences in the field of the viable myocardium.

In the early studies, MCE using intracoronary contrast administration was capable of assessing myocardial perfusion with a potential for predicting myocardial viability as stunning (17) and hybernated myocardium (18). The underlying basis for assessing myocardial viability with MCE is that myocardial contrast enhancement depends on an intact microcirculation. Accordingly, the absence of myocardial opacification with MCE is the evidence of lack of myocardial viability.

Nowadays, this technique utilizes a bolus (or continuous infusion) of specific echocardiographic contrast, injected intravenously. The novel echocardiographic technique uses a low mechanical index to avoid the bubble destruction; it is also possible to visualize the myocardial contrast replenishment after a "flash" imaging with high mechanical index, which destroys the microbubbles in the myocardium.

When comparing different techniques for the evaluation of hibernating myocardium, the use of MCE, rest-redistribution Tl-201 tomography or any contractile reserve shows a high sensitivity with a moderate-to-low specificity for predicting recovery of function (Fig. 13). Importantly, all the above three methods identifies all patients with a significant increase in ejection fraction (Fig. 13) (18).

Recent studies have demonstrated the pathological and vascular correlates of intravenous quantitative MCE parameters in the hibernating myocardium and

Identification of hibernating myocardium: comparative accuracy of MCE, thallium-201, and dobutamine echo

Table Accuracy of Various Modalities in Prediction of Recovery of Function After Revascularization in Severly Dysfunctional Segments

Imaging modality	Sensitivity	Specificity	PPV	NPV	Accuracy
DE (biphasic)	23/34 (68%)*	49/59 (83%)*	23/33 (70%)	49/60 (82%)	72/93 (77%)
DE (any improvement)	31/34 (91%)	39/59 (66%)	31/51 (61%)	39/42 (93%)	70/93 (75%)
MCE (visual score)	41/46 (89%)	32/63 (51%)	41/72 (57%)	32/37 (86%)	73/109 (67%)
MCE ((PI ratio > 0.25)	41/46 (89%)	36/63 (57%)	41/68 (60%)	36/41 (88%)	77/109 (71%)
TI-201 (R-R ≥ 60%)	42/46 (91%)	27/63 (43%)	42/78 (54%)	27/31 (87%)	69/109 (63%)

*$p < 0.01$ versus dobutamine echocardiography, any improvement, thallium-201 and myocardial contrast echocardiography. Data are presented as number (%) of patients. DE, dobutamine echocardiography; MCE, myocardial contrast echocardiography; NPV, negaive predictive value; PI, peak intensity; PPV, positive predictive value; R-R, rest-redistribution; TI-201, thallium-201.

FIGURE 13 Sensitivity and specificity of various imaging modalities in prediction of recovery of myocardial function after revascularization. *Source*: Adapted from Ref. 18.

assessed the predictive value of MCE for the recovery of function of dysfunctional, ischemic myocardium (19).

The MCE has also been useful to demonstrate the beneficial effect of preinfarction angina on viability; in fact this kind of "clinical preconditioning" preserves microvascular integrity and functional vasodilation after AMI, reduces myocardial damage, and favors myocardial viability, limiting left ventricular remodeling (20).

In conclusion, the postinfarction viability is an important pathophysiologic character that needs to be evaluated with dobutamine echocardiography or other cardiac diagnostic tests, in order to better individualize revascularization and medical therapy.

DVD note: The following loops are related to the content of this chapter: 44–50, 68. These loops can be found in the provided DVD.

REFERENCES

1. Bolli R. Myocardial "stunning" in man. Circulation 1992; 86:1671–1691.
2. Rahimtoola SH. The hibernating myocardium. Am Heart J 1989; 117:211–221.
3. Iliceto S, Galiuto L, Colonna P, et al. Functional role of microvascular integrity in patients with infarct related artery patency after acute myocardial infarction. Eur Heart J 1997; 18:618–624.
4. Colonna P, Cadeddu C, Montisci R, et al. Post-infarction microvascular integrity predicts myocardial viability and left ventricular remodeling after primary coronary angioplasty. A study performed with intravenous myocardial contrast echocardiography. Ital Heart J 2002; 3:506–513.
5. Allman KC, Shaw LJ, Hachamovitch R, et al. Myocardial viability testing and impact of revascularization on prognosis in patients with coronary artery disease and left ventricular dysfunction: A meta-analysis. J Am Coll Cardiol 2002; 39:1151–1158.

6. Pierard LA, De Landsheere C, Berthe C, et al. Identification of viable myocardium by echocardiography during dobutamine infusion in patients with myocardial infarction after thrombolytic theraphy: Comparison with positron emission tomography. J Am Coll Cardiol 1990; 15:1021–1031.
7. Bax JJ, Wijns W, Cornel JH, et al. Accuracy of currently available techniques for prediction of functional recovery after revascularization in patients with left ventricular dysfunction due to chronic coronary artery disease: Comparison of pooled data. J Am Coll Cardiol 1997; 30:1451–1460.
8. Smart SC, Sawada S, Ryan T, et al. Low-dose dobutamine echocardiography detects reversible dysfunction after thrombolytic therapy of myocardial infarction. Circulation 1993; 88:405–415.
9. Watada H, Ito H, Oh H, et al. Dobutamine stress echocardiography predicts reversible dysfunction and quantitates the extent of irreversibly damaged myocardium after reperfusion of anterior myocardial infarction. J Am Coll Cardiol 1994; 24:624–630.
10. Sklenar J, Ismail S, Villanueva FS, et al. Dobutamine echocardiography for determining the extent of myocardial salvage after reperfusion: An experimental evaluation. Circulation 1994; 90:1502–1512.
11. Lualdi JC, Douglas PS. Echocardiography for the assessment of myocardial viability. J Am Soc Echocardiogr 1997; 10:772–781.
12. Colonna P, Montisci R, Galiuto L, et al. Effects of acute myocardial ischemia on intramyocardial contraction heterogeneity. A study performed with ultrasound integrated backscatter during transesophageal atrial pacing. Circulation 1999; 100:1770–1776.
13. Lee KS, Marwick TH, Cook SA, et al. Prognosis of patients with left ventricular dysfunction, with and without viable myocardium after myocardial infarction: Relative efficacy of medical therapy and revascularization. Circulation 1994; 90:2687–2694.
14. Tarakji KG, Brunken R, McCarthy PM, et al. Myocardial viability testing and the effect of early intervention in patients with advanced left ventricular systolic dysfunction. Circulation 2006; 113(2): 230–237.
15. Marwick TH, Zuchowski C, Lauer MS, et al. Functional status and quality of life in patients with heart failure undergoing coronary bypass surgery after assessment of myocardial viability. J Am Coll Cardiol 1999; 33:750–758.
16. Meluzin J, Cerny J, Frelich M, et al. Prognostic value of the amount of dysfunctional but viable myocardium in revascularized patients with coronary artery disease and left ventricular dysfunction. JACC 1998; 32:912–920.
17. Iliceto S, Galiuto L, Colonna P, et al. Analysis of microvascular integrity, contractile reserve and myocardial viability after acute myocardial infarction by dobutamine echocardiography and myocardial contrast echocardiography. Am J Cardiol 1996; 77:441–445.
18. Nagueh AF, Vaduganathan P, Ali N, et al. Identification of hibernating myocardium: Comparative accuracy of myocardial contrast echocardiography, rest redistribution thallium-201 tomography and dobutamine echocardiography. JACC 1997; 29:985–993.
19. Shimoni S, Frangogiannis G, Aggeli CJ, et al. Identification of hibernating myocardium with quantitative intravenous myocardial contrast echocardiography. Circulation 2002; 107:538–544.
20. Colonna P, Cadeddu C, Montisci R, et al. Reduced microvascular and myocardial damage in patients with acute myocardial infarction and preinfarction angina. Am Heart J 2002; 144(5):796–803.

8 Contrast in Stress Echocardiography

Navtej S. Chahal and Roxy Senior

Department of Cardiology, Northwick Park Hospital, Harrow, U.K.

I. STRESS ECHOCARDIOGRAPHY AND CONTRAST

Stress echocardiography is a mature, powerful tool for the diagnosis and risk stratification of patients with coronary artery disease. Advances in imaging technology have ensured that previous misgivings concerning endocardial border delineation and reproducibility have been largely overcome. Although tissue harmonic imaging has helped to reduce interobserver variability and improve the sensitivity of stress echocardiography (1,2), left ventricular opacification (LVO) with ultrasonic contrast still confers a benefit over harmonic imaging during stress echocardiography. Furthermore, with the combined evolution of contrast agents and imaging technology simultaneous evaluation of LV structure, function, and perfusion is now feasible at the bedside.

Contrast echocardiography enables enhanced discrimination between myocardial tissue and the blood pool by opacifying the LV cavity and at the same time making the myocardium appear dark (Fig. 1).

A. Contrast Agents

Left ventricular opacification is achieved using microbubbles. An engineered microbubble comprises a gas contained by an outer shell and these constituents determine the reflective characteristics, duration of contrast, and biological activity. Bubble shells can be designed to be either rigid or flexible and to have varying resistance to collapse at high pressure. Manipulation of these characteristics can allow the creation of microbubbles that either persist for a longer time in the circulation thereby providing longer contrast effect, or bubbles that are easily destroyed in the ultrasound beam, resulting in simulated acoustic emission and enhanced detectability by this mechanism.

Early contrast agents were air-filled microbubbles which were relatively unstable and incapable of withstanding transpulmonary passage, making them unsuitable for opacification of left-sided structures. Therefore, second-generation agents were developed containing a gas with low solubility and diffusivity encapsulated by a shell of lipids, albumin, or galactose to improve their longevity. These new microbubbles are smaller than a red blood cell, resist arterial pressure, and remain intact after passage through the pulmonary vasculature. The most used commercially available second-generation agents available today are SonoVue, Luminity, and Optison (Table 1).

In general microbubbles generate echo contrast by increasing backscatter in an ultrasound field. The nature of backscatter is related to the degree of microbubble contraction and expansion (oscillation), which in turn is affected by the acoustic power of the transmitted ultrasound field or the mechanical index (MI). With low MI imaging (<0.1), microbubbles demonstrate linear oscillations

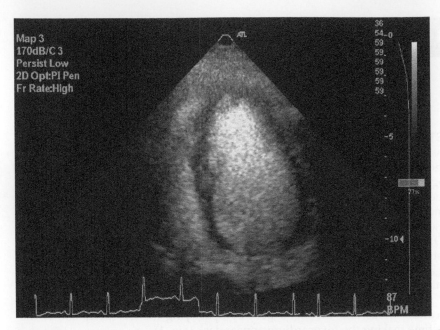

Map 3
170dB/C 3
Persist Low
2D Opt:PI Pen
Fr Rate:High

36
54 0
59
59
59
59
59
59

-5

-10

87
BPM

FIGURE 1 Improved delineation of the interface between blood and endothelium achieved with contrast agents (loop 51).

where contraction and expansion of the bubble are equal (loop 52). All returning backscatter remains within the range of the frequency transmitted by the transducer (the fundamental frequency). Intermediate MI imaging (0.1–0.3) generates nonlinear oscillations whereby expansion is greater than contraction and the microbubble produces backscatter of low amplitude, second harmonic frequencies (loop 53).

When a microbubble is exposed to high mechanical index imaging (MI > 0.6; as in standard imaging), the bubbles oscillate wildly and burst (loop 54). Upon destruction a subpopulation of smaller bubbles are produced which have a broad range of resonant frequencies rich in harmonic signals. Even after bubble destruction, high-density perfluorocarbons that diffuse more slowly from the blood pool can also provide brief contrast effect. Importantly at high MI, tissues also produce harmonics, therefore, the aim is to enhance the contrast to tissue

TABLE 1 Characteristics of Currently Available Second-Generation Microbubble Contrast Agents

	SonoVue	Optison	Luminity (Definity in the U.S.A.)
Gas	Sulfur hexafluoride	Perfluoropropane	Perfluoropropane
Mean bubble size (μm)	2–8	3.0–4.5	1.1–2.5
Shell composition	Predominantly phospholipid	Human albumin	Predominantly phospholipid
Manufacturer	Bracco	GE	Bristol-Myers Squibb

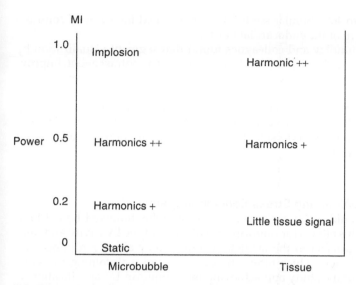

FIGURE 2 Intermediate MI harmonic imaging allows high frame rate imaging, results in reduced bubble destruction and leads to production of microbubble harmonic signals with minimal tissue harmonics and maximal discrimination between blood pool and tissue.

backscatter signal ratio to achieve optimal endocardial delineation during LVO (Fig. 2).

II. ENHANCED ENDOCARDIAL BORDER DELINEATION WITH CONTRAST ECHOCARDIOGRAPHY

Approximately 20% of resting echocardiograms using fundamental imaging inadequately define the endocardium (3). This problem seems to be worse in patients referred for stress echocardiography, with as many as 33% reported as having poor visualization of the endocardial borders (4,5). Although tissue harmonic imaging provides better endocardial delineation, 5% to 10% of patients still have suboptimal studies (5). Obesity, chronic lung disease, ventilatory support, and chest wall deformities may impair image quality thus limit reader confidence, decrease diagnostic accuracy, and result in poor reproducibility (6).

Sonicated human serum albumin (Albunex, Molecular Biosystems, CA) was the first agent approved for the role of LVO in 1992 by the FDA. However, consistent LVO was difficult with this agent largely because of its fragility and short duration of effect of the air-containing microbubble. In patients with low cardiac output states, significant LVO was observed in <50%.

Second-generation agents have subsequently been shown to achieve diagnostic quality images more reliably. A multicenter study of more than 200 patients in whom LVO was achieved with Optison (Molecular Biosystems) demonstrated enhanced degree of LVO, number, and length of LV endocardial border segments visualized and duration of enhancement to be superior to Albunex (7). Contrast administration transformed 75% of previous nondiagnostic studies to a diagnostic echocardiogram with diagnostic information increasing by 35% to 40%. Similar studies have confirmed the value of contrast-enhanced assessment of the endocardial border (8).

A study by Hundley and colleagues found that segment visualization by echo was comparable to MRI after the administration of a contrast agent, improving from 86% to 99% of segments visualized (9). In particular, visualization of the anterior and lateral walls was observed with contrast, as was the detection of segments with abnormal wall motion. A significant improvement in interobserver agreement for visualization of the endocardium, determination of normal versus abnormal wall motion, and assessment of regional wall motion was also found with the use of contrast.

A. Protocol for LVO During Stress Echocardiography

Contrast agents should be administered as a slow bolus followed by a 10-mL slow saline flush. This allows for uniform opacification of the LV cavity and minimizes attenuation artefact in the far-field. Contrast may also be administered as a continuous infusion, which offers the advantage of maintaining the same flow rate throughout the study and achieving more uniform LV opacification as compared to bolus injections.

Typically the mechanical index used should be intermediate (0.4–0.5) (loop 55), however, low-power imaging (MI 0.1–0.2) allows simultaneous assessment of function and perfusion, and in conjunction with high-sensitivity ultrasonography systems requires less volume of contrast to be administered (loop 56).

B. Stress Echocardiography with LVO

Myocardial ischemia manifests during stress echocardiography as the occurrence of reduced systolic wall thickening when myocardial oxygen demand exceeds myocardial blood supply. For stress echocardiography to be feasible, accurate evaluation of regional systolic wall thickening is essential and largely dependent on adequate endocardial border resolution.

Conventional stress echocardiography is well established with a high sensitivity and specificity for the diagnosis of coronary artery disease (CAD). However, endocardial visualization can be compromised during stress echocardiography by chest wall movement during hyperventilation (with exercise stress) and cardiac translational movement during tachycardia. Poor-quality studies have been shown to be less reproducible and to have low interobserver agreement (10). Moreover, quick and reliable acquisition of diagnostic quality images is mandated during stress echocardiography, particularly when exercise stress is undertaken.

The benefit of ultrasonic contrast agents in endocardial delineation during stress studies has been unequivocally confirmed. Early studies using sonicated albumin demonstrated improved wall motion scoring and reproducibility during stress echocardiography (11). Second-generation contrast agents have shown improved endocardial resolution, greater concordance in test interpretation, and greater confidence in wall motion analysis even by less-experienced readers (12–14) (Fig. 3).

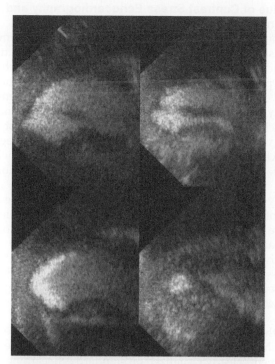

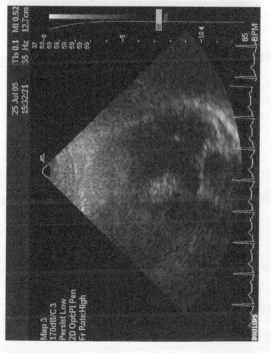

FIGURE 3 Rest imaging performed without contrast (loop 57) and stress echocardiography performed with LV opacification (loop 58). With LV opacification there is a clear benefit for endocardial border detection, demonstrating a defect in wall motion at rest and during stress.

C.   Diagnostic Value of Contrast Stress Echocardiography and Cost-Effectiveness

There has been a relative paucity of studies demonstrating the incremental value of contrast during stress echocardiography on the diagnostic accuracy of the test. Dolan et al. studied 229 patients of which 117 had poor rest echocardiography and received Optison during dobutamine stress echo, while the remainder were deemed to have adequate rest images not requiring contrast enhancement. Optison significantly improved endocardial border visualization, and the ability to measure wall thickening was significantly higher in the contrast group with suboptimal images versus the noncontrast group with optimal images (89% vs. 71%, $p = 0.01$), which resulted in comparable sensitivity and specificity between the groups in the diagnosis of significant CAD on subsequent angiography (15) (Fig. 4).

A recent study by Moir and colleagues assessed whether the routine use of LVO, regardless of baseline image quality, would provide incremental benefit and be cost-effective for the diagnosis of CAD. Contrast echocardiography was performed in 185 patients referred for coronary angiography. LVO significantly increased the sensitivity of stress echocardiography from 80% to 91% ($p = 0.03$), including single vessel disease, with no significant change in specificity. Loop 61 exemplifies how even subtle wall motion abnormalities due to single-vessel disease can be diagnosed. This patient had a significant stenosis of the posterior descending artery.

Interestingly there was no relationship between resting image quality and diagnostic benefit when using LVO, with 42% (8/19) patients who benefited from LVO having all segments clearly visualized on standard echocardiography. However, despite the diagnostic benefit of using LVO in all patients irrespective of the quality of endocardial delineation at rest, such a strategy did not prove cost-effective as the downstream risks associated with a false-negative scan in a typical patient with benign stable angina tend not to be high (16).

When contrast is used judiciously for LVO during stress echocardiography, it has been demonstrated to be cost-effective. One study showed that the improved diagnostic yield achieved with contrast-enhanced stress echocardiography resulted in only 12% of patients requiring further down-stream testing, compared with 42% of patients who received unenhanced stress scans (17). Thanigaraj et al. (4) defined the cost-effectiveness of contrast usage in patients with suboptimal image quality during stress echocardiography with respect to its influence on further cost incurred for the same clinical indication. During a 3-week period after stress echocardiography, 53% of patients who underwent suboptimal, unenhanced scans (due to patient declining contrast injection or contraindication to contrast administration) required additional testing in the form of nuclear scintigraphy. This compared to only 3% requiring additional nuclear stress testing in the contrast-enhanced stress echocardiography group ($p < 0.0001$).

III.   MYOCARDIAL PERFUSION CONTRAST

Detection and quantification of myocardial perfusion have been goals of echocardiography since LVO was first achieved reliably. In the ischemic cascade, it has been well established that abnormalities of myocardial perfusion precede those of wall motion which precede ECG changes (18). Techniques that image

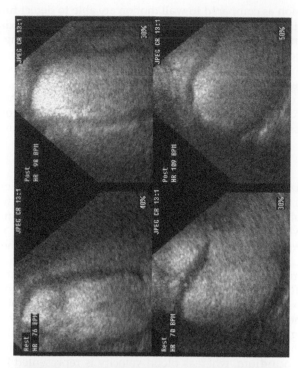

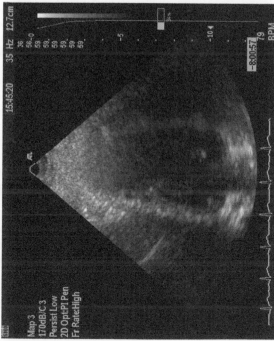

FIGURE 4 Interpretation of LV wall motion and function was difficult at rest with unenhanced echocardiography (loop 59), however, following stress echocardiography with LVO inducible ischemia in the LAD territory and cavity dilatation was demonstrated (loop 60).

myocardial perfusion as compared to wall motion are able to detect functionally significant CAD at an earlier stage of stress and potentially at submaximal stress (19). Single-photon emission computed tomography (SPECT) imaging is a well-established method for the diagnosis of CAD and prediction of outcomes. However, there are technical limitations with SPECT and the technique also involves radiation exposure as well as being costly.

Myocardial contrast echocardiography (MCE) allows real-time quantification of myocardial perfusion and can be performed simultaneously with conventional stress echocardiography, thereby enhancing the sensitivity of the procedure.

A. Physiology

Clinical MCE utilizes the unique physical features of second-generation contrast ultrasound agents to provide a physiological method of assessing perfusion. The gas-filled microbubbles possess a rheology (mechanical behavior) similar to red blood cells and whereas MRI tracers diffuse into the extravascular space and radionuclides enter myocytes, microbubbles remain entirely within the intravascular space.

The blood present within the coronary microcirculation constitutes approximately 8% of left ventricular mass and is termed myocardial blood volume (MBV). As approximately 90% of the total MBV lies within the capillaries, the opacification of the myocardium that is seen during MCE essentially represents blood flow through the capillaries. This myocardial blood flow is the product of MBV and red blood cell velocity. MBV is directly related to the intensity of contrast in the myocardium, whereas blood velocity is represented by the rate of increase of intensity after bubble destruction. In the absence of a significant coronary stenosis, coronary flow during stress can increase by a factor of 4 to 6-fold to meet oxygen demand. This is achieved through a process of coronary autoregulation, principally mediated by vasodilatation of the arterioles. In the presence of a noncritical (60–90%) stenosis, resting MBF and systolic wall thickening remain normal due to resting arteriolar vasodilatation. During stress, however, this mechanism is quickly exhausted and capillaries are derecruited in order to maintain adequate transcapillary pressure revealing a perfusion mismatch.

Therefore, determination of MBF reserve when using MCE is important in patients with noncritical lesions to quantify the degree of ischemia. As mentioned previously, during maximal hyperemia coronary flow reserve is in the order of 4 to 6 times greater than at rest in normal, unobstructed arteries. As MCE can quantify resting and hyperemic blood flow, MBF reserve can be derived quantitatively using this technique.

B. Assessment of Myocardial Perfusion

Perfusion can be measured qualitatively by assessing the signal intensity, pattern of filling, and rate of filling of myocardial contrast opacification.

Qualitative Assessment

During continuous infusion of microbubbles in a patient with intact coronary microvasculature and normal MBF, destruction of the microbubbles in the microcirculation by ultrasound is followed by the relatively uniform appearance of contrast in the coronary microcirculation and homogenous opacification of the

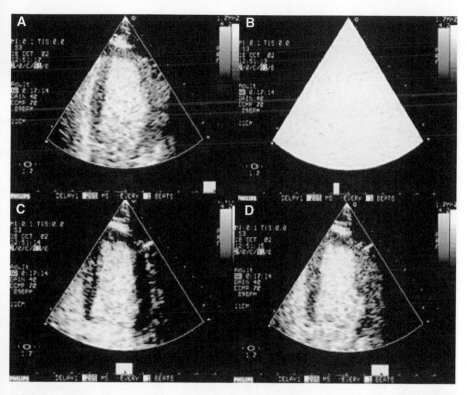

FIGURE 5 Destruction replenishment imaging with real-time MCE during hyperemia (loop 63). (**A**) 1 beat preflash, (**B**) flash delivered, (**C**) 1 beat postflash, and (**D**) 2 beats postflash with normal, homogenous opacification of the myocardium demonstrated.

myocardium. In the case of diminished epicardial flow in patients with significant CAD, the speed of contrast replenishment and the signal intensity that represents MBV are diminished. Signal intensity can be quantified using a graded scale reflecting homogenous perfusion, reduced perfusion, and absent perfusion. At rest the RBC velocity in capillaries is 1 mm/sec; therefore, following destruction of microbubbles in the myocardium, it takes approximately 5 seconds (at resting heart rate 60–80 seconds) to replenish an ultrasound beam of 5-mm elevation (loop 62). In the presence of hyperemia, without coronary stenosis, myocardial blood flow should increase 4 to 6-fold and homogenous myocardial perfusion within 1 to 2 seconds (Fig. 5). In regions of coronary stenosis, rate of filling is much slower depending on the severity of stenosis (Fig. 6).

The distribution of perfusion in relation to the extent of myocardium involved is also important in being able to confidently diagnose ischemia qualitatively. Stress-induced ischemia tends to cause perfusion defects restricted to the subendocardium, whereas transmural or epicardial defects are more likely to represent artefact. Such subendocardial defects can be missed on radionuclide imaging which has poorer resolution than MCE (20) (Fig. 7).

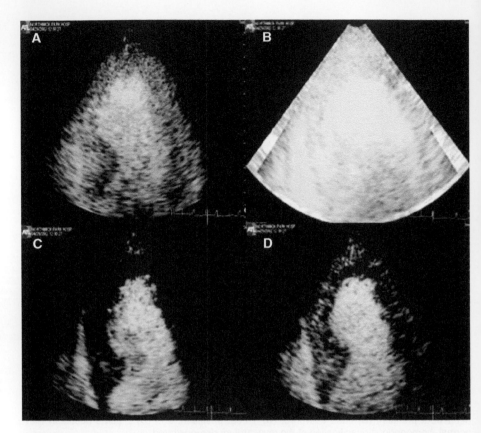

FIGURE 6 A clear perfusion defect is seen following vasodilator stress which persists 3 beats after microbubble destruction (**D**) extending from the mid-septum to the entire lateral wall (loop 64). This patient had 70% LAD stenosis and occlusion of the circumflex artery on subsequent coronary angiography.

Quantitative Assessment

The replenishment of contrast after microbubble destruction can be characterized by a time-intensity curve from which MBF can be determined. Animal studies using a coronary stenosis model have demonstrated that MBF estimated by MCE correlates with absolute MBF measured with radiolabeled fluorescent microspheres (21,22). In humans, abnormalities in MBF reserve have been used to quantify stenosis severity (23).

C. Protocol for the Assessment of Function and Perfusion by Stress Echocardiography

The authors prefer continuous infusion of the contrast agent, as this allows a steady state to be reached which is a prerequisite for accurate assessment of myocardial perfusion. Low-power mechanical index imaging (0.1–0.2) permits real-time assessment of function and perfusion simultaneously. Figure 8 illustrates the protocol utilized in our laboratory.

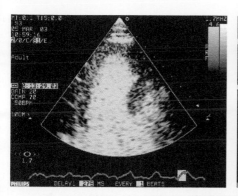
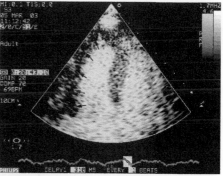
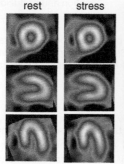
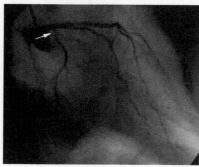

rest   stress

FIGURE 7 (*See color insert*) MCE on a patient at rest (*left*, loop 65) and with stress (*right*, loop 66). There is a clear subendocardial perfusion defect in the circumflex artery territory (*black arrows*). Radionuclide uptake on SPECT was normal. Coronary angiography confirmed the presence of a flow-limiting lesion in the circumflex artery (loop 67).

D. Stress Echocardiography and MCE

As reduction in blood flow precedes reduction in myocardial thickening during the ischemic cascade, assessment of perfusion simultaneous to wall motion analysis should theoretically provide greater sensitivity for the diagnosis of CAD during stress echocardiography. A number of studies have established an incremental role of perfusion imaging over wall motion analysis alone in patients undergoing stress echocardiography. In a study by Xie et al. (24), two separate stress echo studies were performed in patients who presented with chest pain. The first study involved dobutamine stress without contrast to analyze wall motion followed by a contrast study to assess perfusion and wall motion, again with dobutamine. Twenty-one of the 27 patients had significant CAD on subsequent coronary angiography, 14 of which had abnormal perfusion detected at peak stress and 7 had abnormal wall motion detected by standard stress echocardiography.

Porter et al. performed MCE in 117 patients during DSE. Regional myocardial contrast defects at stress were observed in 30 patients with >50% stenosis in at least one vessel (13 with single-vessel and 17 with multivessel disease, total

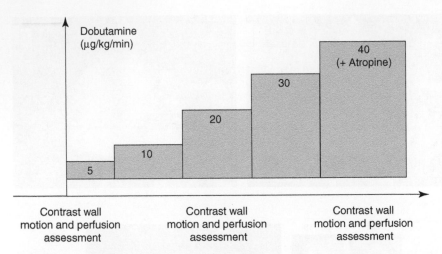

FIGURE 8 Protocol for assessment of wall motion and perfusion. Loop 68 illustrates normal perfusion at rest and during stress with dobutamine. Loop 69 is an example of a transmural apical perfusion defect diagnosed following myocardial contrast echocardiography using an exercise stress protocol.

of 55 coronary artery territories). Contrast defects were observed at peak stress in 46 (84%) of the 55 territories. Although wall motion and contrast enhancement were in agreement in 90% of the coronary artery territories, there was a significant number of territories subtended by a >50% stenosis, which exhibited contrast defects despite normal wall motion. The overall concordance between MCE and quantitative angiography was 83%, compared to 72% for wall motion analysis and angiography (25).

Experimental studies have shown that myocardial perfusion abnormalities precede wall motion abnormalities during dobutamine infusion and that assessment of myocardial perfusion may potentially improve the sensitivity of DSE in patients with submaximal stress (18). This temporal sequence of events has been confirmed clinically in a study that sought to compare the accuracy of MCE and wall motion analysis during submaximal and peak DSE for the diagnosis of CAD (19). The authors found that the majority of inducible perfusion abnormalities occur at an intermediate phase of stress without wall motion abnormalities and that MCE had a higher sensitivity compared to wall motion abnormalities at maximal stress (91% vs. 70%) and intermediate stress (84% vs. 20%) for the detection of CAD.

E. Limitations of MCE with Stress Echocardiography

It has been shown that MCE has a lower specificity for the diagnosis of CAD as compared to wall motion analysis (26). This is because impairment of myocardial perfusion and coronary flow reserve may occur in various other conditions such as hypertension, diabetes, and left ventricular hypertrophy. However, the presence of a subendocardial defect is almost certainly due to flow-limiting CAD.

IV. CONCLUSIONS

The enhanced diagnostic accuracy conferred by ultrasound contrast agents has made them indispensible in the day-to-day performance of stress echocardiography. Advances in microbubble and imaging technology have permitted qualitative and quantitative assessment of myocardial perfusion, further improving the sensitivity of stress echocardiography in the detection of CAD.

> **DVD note:** The following loops are related to the content of this chapter: 51–69. These loops can be found in the provided DVD.

REFERENCES

1. Becher H, Tiemann K, Schlosser T, et al. Improvement in endocardial border delineation using tissue harmonic imaging. Echocardiography 1998; 15:511–518.
2. Senior R, Soman P, Khattar RS, et al. Improved endocardial visualization with second harmonic imaging compared with fundamental two-dimensional echocardiographic imaging. Am Heart J 1999; 138:163–168.
3. Schiller NB, Shah PM, Crawford M, et al. Recommendations for quantitation of the left ventricle by two-dimensional echocardiography. American Society of Echocardiography Committee on Standards, Subcommittee on Quantitation of Two-Dimensional Echocardiograms. J Am Soc Echocardiogr 1989; 2:358–367.
4. Thanigaraj S, Nease RF Jr, Schechtman KB, et al. Use of contrast for image enhancement during stress echocardiography is cost-effective and reduces additional diagnostic testing. Am J Cardiol 2001; 87:1430–1432.
5. Hoffmann R, Marwick TH, Poldermans D, et al. Refinements in stress echocardiographic techniques improve inter-institutional agreement in interpretation of dobutamine stress echocardiograms. Eur Heart J 2002; 23:821–829.
6. Yong Y, Wu D, Fernandes V, et al. Diagnostic accuracy and cost-effectiveness of contrast echocardiography on evaluation of cardiac function in technically very difficult patients in the intensive care unit. Am J Cardiol 2002; 89:711–718.
7. Cohen JL, Cheirif J, Segar DS, et al. Improved left ventricular endocardial border delineation and opacification with OPTISON (FS069), a new echocardiographic contrast agent. Results of a phase III Multicenter Trial. J Am Coll Cardiol 1998; 32:746–752.
8. Grayburn PA, Weiss JL, Hack TC, et al. Phase III multicenter trial comparing the efficacy of 2% dodecafluoropentane emulsion (EchoGen) and sonicated 5% human albumin (Albunex) as ultrasound contrast agents in patients with suboptimal echocardiograms. J Am Coll Cardiol 1998; 32:230–236.
9. Hundley WG, Kizilbash AM, Afridi I, et al. Administration of an intravenous perfluorocarbon contrast agent improves echocardiographic determination of left ventricular volumes and ejection fraction: Comparison with cine magnetic resonance imaging. J Am Coll Cardiol 1998; 32:1426–1432.
10. Hoffmann R, Lethen H, Marwick T, et al. Standardized guidelines for the interpretation of dobutamine echocardiography reduce interinstitutional variance in interpretation. Am J Cardiol 1998; 82:1520–1524.
11. Porter TR, Xie F, Kricsfeld A, et al. Improved endocardial border resolution during dobutamine stress echocardiography with intravenous sonicated dextrose albumin. J Am Coll Cardiol 1994; 23:1440–1443.
12. Ikonomidis I, Holmes E, Narbuvold H, et al. Assessment of left ventricular wall motion and delineation of the endocardial border after intravenous injection of Infoson during dobutamine stress echocardiography. Coron Artery Dis 1998; 9:567–576.
13. Malhotra V, Nwogu J, Bondmass MD, et al. Is the technically limited echocardiographic study an endangered species? Endocardial border definition with native tissue harmonic imaging and Optison contrast: A review of 200 cases. J Am Soc Echocardiogr 2000; 13:771–773.

14. Rainbird AJ, Mulvagh SL, Oh JK, et al. Contrast dobutamine stress echocardiography: Clinical practice assessment in 300 consecutive patients. J Am Soc Echocardiogr 2001; 14:378–385.
15. Dolan MS, Riad K, El-Shafei A, et al. Effect of intravenous contrast for left ventricular opacification and border definition on sensitivity and specificity of dobutamine stress echocardiography compared with coronary angiography in technically difficult patients. Am Heart J 2001; 142:908–915.
16. Moir S, Shaw L, Haluska B, et al. Left ventricular opacification for the diagnosis of coronary artery disease with stress echocardiography: An angiographic study of incremental benefit and cost-effectiveness. Am Heart J 2007; 154:510–518.
17. Shaw LJ, Gillam L, Feinstein S, et al. Use of an intravenous contrast agent (Optison) to enhance echocardiography: Efficacy and cost implications. Optison Multicenter Study Group. Am J Manag Care 1998; 4(Spec No.):SP169–SP176.
18. Leong-Poi H, Rim SJ, Le DE, et al. Perfusion versus function: The ischemic cascade in demand ischemia: Implications of single-vessel versus multivessel stenosis. Circulation 2002; 105:987–992.
19. Elhendy A, Geleijnse ML, Roelandt JR, et al. Dobutamine-induced hypoperfusion without transient wall motion abnormalities: Less severe ischemia or less severe stress? J Am Coll Cardiol 1996; 27:323–329.
20. Senior R, Lepper W, Pasquet A, et al. Myocardial perfusion assessment in patients with medium probability of coronary artery disease and no prior myocardial infarction: Comparison of myocardial contrast echocardiography with 99mTc single-photon emission computed tomography. Am Heart J 2004; 147:1100–1105.
21. Masugata H, Lafitte S, Peters B, et al. Comparison of real-time and intermittent triggered myocardial contrast echocardiography for quantification of coronary stenosis severity and transmural perfusion gradient. Circulation 2001; 104:1550–1556.
22. Wei K, Jayaweera AR, Firoozan S, et al. Quantification of myocardial blood flow with ultrasound-induced destruction of microbubbles administered as a constant venous infusion. Circulation 1998; 97:473–483.
23. Wei K, Ragosta M, Thorpe J, et al. Noninvasive quantification of coronary blood flow reserve in humans using myocardial contrast echocardiography. Circulation 2001; 103:2560–2565.
24. Xie F, Tsutsui JM, McGrain AC, et al. Comparison of dobutamine stress echocardiography with and without real-time perfusion imaging for detection of coronary artery disease. Am J Cardiol 2005; 96:506–511.
25. Porter TR, Xie F, Silver M, et al. Real-time perfusion imaging with low mechanical index pulse inversion Doppler imaging. J Am Coll Cardiol 2001; 37:748–753.
26. Elhendy A, O'Leary EL, Xie F, et al. Comparative accuracy of real-time myocardial contrast perfusion imaging and wall motion analysis during dobutamine stress echocardiography for the diagnosis of coronary artery disease. J Am Coll Cardiol 2004; 44:2185–2191.

9 Stress Testing in Valvular Heart Disease

Leonardo Rodriguez

Cardiovascular Imaging Center, Heart and Vascular Institute, Cleveland Clinic, Cleveland, Ohio, U.S.A.

Valvular heart disease is an important field in cardiovascular medicine. Traditionally, patients are presented to the clinician because of their symptoms. With the widespread use of echocardiography, valvular heart disease is often detected long before symptoms appear and the important issue of timing of surgery has become a controversial one. While the presence of symptoms or left ventricular dysfunction is still the main factor to be considered for surgical indication, additional parameters may also be relevant.

Stress test is an important tool in the evaluation of patients with structural heart disease. It can objectively assess functional capacity, elicit symptoms, and uncover latent ventricular dysfunction and pulmonary hypertension with exercise. In some cases, a valvular lesion that appears only moderate at rest may show significant hemodynamic importance with exercise.

The guidelines published by the American College of Cardiology/American Heart Association (ACC/AHA) (1), the European Society of Cardiology (ESC) (2), and the American Society of Echocardiography (ASE) (3) mention the role of stress testing in valvular heart disease and its application in specific valvular lesions.

Stress echo laboratories need to be familiar with patients with valvular heart disease and adapt their protocols to answer specific questions in this population. Both treadmill and bicycle ergometry have been utilized. Each one has its own advantages and its use should be based in individual expertise. Dobutamine echocardiography is used predominantly in patients with aortic stenosis and left ventricular dysfunction.

Patient selection is of crucial importance. Stress test is safe in asymptomatic or minimally symptomatic patients, but should not be performed in patients with severe valvular disease and overt symptoms.

I. AORTIC VALVE

A. Aortic Stenosis

In the majority of patients, the indication for surgery can be done based on the clinical and hemodynamic parameters (1,2). However, stress test can be very useful in asymptomatic patients, in those with questionable symptoms, and also in determining prognosis when advanced ventricular dysfunction is present.

In asymptomatic patients, the purpose of the test is to unmask symptoms or an abnormal hemodynamic response (i.e., decrease in blood pressure). The presence of abnormal electrocardiographic findings has also been reported as an important prognosticator. The relative importance of these parameters is

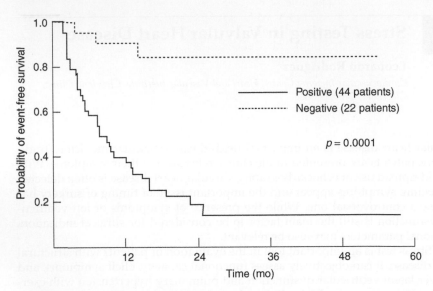

FIGURE 1 Kaplan–Meier life table analysis for probability of event-free survival over 60 months for patients with asymptomatic severe aortic stenosis, according to positive or negative results of exercise testing. *Source*: From Ref. 5.

controversial. In asymptomatic patients, Otto et al. found that exercise parameters have no additional value over jet velocity, rate of change in jet velocity over time, and baseline functional status (4). However, the same authors stressed the importance of drop in blood pressure, ST changes, and ventricular arrhythmias during the test. Amato et al. (5) reported an unfavorable prognosis (sudden death or symptoms) in patients with an abnormal stress test defined when one or more of the following were present: symptoms, ST changes, complex arrhythmias, or abnormal blood pressure response (Fig. 1). Using similar criteria, Lancellotti et al. not only reported comparable results but also found that an increase in mean transaortic pressure gradient by ≥18 mm Hg during exercise had incremental prognostic value (6) (Fig. 2). In contrast, Das et al. reported that exercise-limiting symptoms were the only independent predictors of outcome (symptom-free survival) at 12 months, and an abnormal blood pressure response or ST-segment depression did not improve the accuracy of the exercise test (7). The discrepancies may be explained by the different outcomes selected in the studies.

The ACC/AHA guidelines give a class IIb indication to exercise testing in asymptomatic patients with aortic stenosis. The ESC guidelines have a different approach and relate the different stress test responses to the indications for aortic valve replacement.

Aortic valve replacement is indicated in

- asymptomatic patients with severe aortic stenosis and abnormal exercise test showing symptoms on exercise—IC,
- asymptomatic patients with severe aortic stenosis and abnormal exercise test showing fall in blood pressure below baseline—IIaC, or
- asymptomatic patients with severe aortic stenosis and abnormal exercise test showing complex ventricular arrhythmias—IIbC

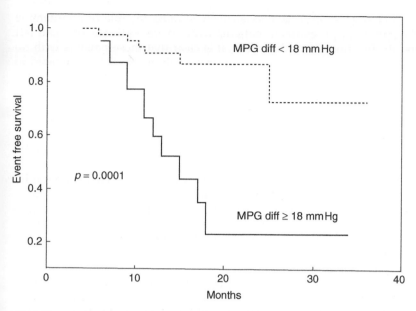

FIGURE 2 Survival curves according to exercise-induced changes in mean transaortic pressure gradient. *Abbreviations*: diff, difference exercise vs. rest; MPG, mean transaortic pressure gradient. *Source*: From Ref. 6.

B. Aortic Stenosis with Left Ventricular Dysfunction

Patients with severe aortic stenosis usually present with normal or hyperdynamic left ventricular function. Some patients, however, have profound systolic dysfunction at the time of diagnosis. This can be the result of associated coronary disease or primary contractile dysfunction. Two important clinical questions are associated with this condition. First, is the reduced valve area due to true calcific stenosis or is it the result of low stroke volume and reduced opening forces? The second question pertains to the operative mortality and long-term prognosis.

Patients with left ventricular dysfunction and high gradients do not present a major diagnostic or therapeutic dilemma. In contrast, the rare patient with low-flow/low-gradient aortic stenosis and left ventricular dysfunction represents a formidable challenge.

Dobutamine echocardiography is an important tool in the diagnosis and management of these patients (8–17). Dobutamine echo protocol is usually started at 5 µg/kg/min and increase up to 20 µg/kg/min. Criteria for terminating the test are reaching maximal dose or an increase in heart rate >10 to 20 beats per minute. At each stage, left ventricular outflow tract and peak aortic velocities should be obtained and aortic valve area calculated. If dobutamine infusion augments valve area more than 0.2 cm^2 (final valve area ≥1 cm^2) with little change in gradient, then the patient most likely does not have severe aortic stenosis. On the contrary, patients with severe aortic stenosis will show a fixed valve area with increasing gradients (loops 70a–b). Patients with no inotropic response to dobutamine remain a diagnostic challenge and other parameters such as degree of valvular calcification need to be taken into account.

Monin et al. (13–15,18) have extensively studied the role of dobutamine echocardiography for prognosis in patients with severe aortic stenosis and left ventricular dysfunction. From their data, it is clear that those patients with no or minimal contractile reserve (increase in stroke volume of <20% compared to baseline values) have a poor prognosis. In particular, there is a striking difference in surgical mortality (6% vs. 33%) (19). However, in those who survive surgery, ejection fraction improves in the majority of patients with low-gradient aortic stenosis. Therefore, the authors recommend that surgery should not be contraindicated on the basis of the absence of contractile reserve alone (19). Bermejo and Yotti (8) elegantly reviewed the limitations of dobutamine echocardiography in patients with left ventricular dysfunction and low flow aortic stenosis.

The ACC/AHA gives a IIaB indication for dobutamine echocardiography in patients with aortic stenosis and left ventricular dysfunction. In the ESC guidelines, patients with aortic stenosis, low gradient (<40 mm Hg), and left ventricular dysfunction with contractile reserve have a IIaC indication for aortic valve surgery and without contractile reserve have a IIbC indication.

C. Aortic Regurgitation

Data on stress echocardiography in patients with severe aortic regurgitation are scarce and the role of this technique in these patients remains unclear. The ESC guidelines state, "clinical decisions should not be based on changes in ejection fraction on exercise, nor on data from stress echocardiography because these indices, although potentially interesting, have not been adequately validated." The ACC/AHA guidelines consider exercise stress testing reasonable for assessment of functional capacity and symptomatic response in patients with a history of equivocal symptoms, and in asymptomatic patients before participation in athletic activities (class IIa indication).

Patients with severe aortic regurgitation undergoing exercise echo may have significant changes in ejection fraction with increased left ventricular systolic volume. Changes in wall motion can be regional even in the absence of coronary artery disease (20), something to keep in mind while interpreting these tests.

Wahi and Marwick (21) showed in a small group of patients that those with contractile reserve (increase in ejection fraction with exercise) have better ejection fraction postoperatively. In those patients treated medically, contractile reserve also predicted changes in ejection fraction at follow-up (Fig. 3). Other prognostic parameters such as fractional shortening and wall stress after exercise has also been reported in small group of patients and need further validation (22).

In our practice, we still use stress test in selected patients, mainly for evaluation of symptoms. In patients with borderline indications for surgery on clinical grounds, a fall in ejection fraction with exercise may tip the balance in favor of surgery, although this approach has not been well validated in clinical trials.

II. MITRAL VALVE

A. Mitral Regurgitation

Patients with severe mitral regurgitation have an indication for surgery when they have symptoms or evidence of left ventricular dysfunction. Reduction of resting ejection fraction is relatively a late event that has been associated with

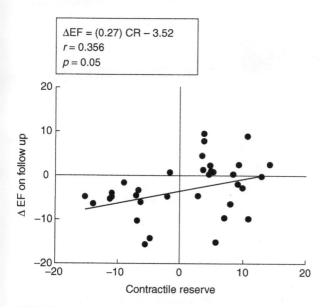

$\Delta EF = (0.27)\ CR - 3.52$
$r = 0.356$
$p = 0.05$

FIGURE 3 Correlation of contractile reserve with change of ejection fraction on follow up in patients with severe aortic regurgitation treated medically. *Abbreviations*: EF, ejection fraction; CR, contractile reserve. *Source*: From Ref. 21.

poor prognosis. Patients with severe mitral regurgitation may have subclinical left ventricular dysfunction not evident by resting parameters. Therefore, stress echocardiography is an attractive technique to evaluate the response of left ventricular size and function to exercise and unmask latent dysfunction (loops 71a–c). In patients with organic mitral regurgitation, the normal left ventricular response to exercise is a decrease in left ventricular systolic volume and increase in ejection fraction. In patients with latent left ventricular dysfunction, there is an increase in end-systolic volume and decrease in ejection fraction with exercise. Leung et at. (23) studied a group of 139 patients with severe mitral regurgitation. Stress echocardiography was performed and end-systolic volume and ejection fraction were calculated before and after treadmill exercise. Absence of contractile reserve (increase in ejection fraction <4%) and an end-systolic volume index >25 mL/m² predicted postoperative left ventricular dysfunction (Fig. 4). Lee et al. (24) used a similar protocol to study 71 patients and follow up them for 3 years. Again, lack of contractile reserved predicted lower event-free survival after surgery (Fig. 5). In medically treated patients those without contractile reserve had progressively lower EF and functional capacity.

Use of tissue Doppler assessment of longitudinal contraction (25) and strain rate have also been proposed to identify contractile reserve. According to the authors, strain rate has the potential to independently predict contractile reserve, with an accuracy superior to that of exercise left ventricular end-systolic volume (26). Although promising, these techniques need further validation.

The ACC/AHA gives a class IIa indication for stress test in asymptomatic severe mitral regurgitation to assess exercise tolerance and the effects of exercise on pulmonary artery pressure and mitral regurgitation severity. Patients with

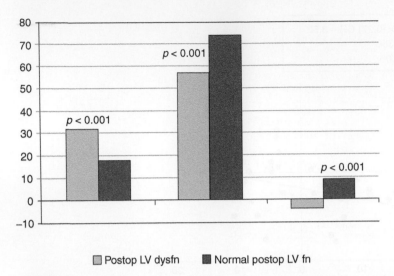

☐ Postop LV dysfn   ■ Normal postop LV fn

FIGURE 4 Compared with patients with normal post mitral valve repair LV function, patients with postoperative LV dysfunction have significantly larger preoperative exercise end-systolic volume index (left bars), lower exercise ejection fraction (middle bars), and lower change in ejection fraction with exercise (right bars), *Abbreviations:* LV dysfn, left ventricular dysfunction; LV fn, left ventricular function; postop, postoperative. *Source*: From Ref. 23.

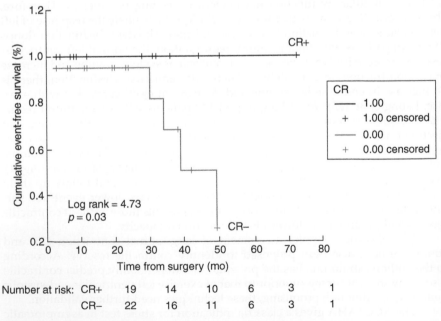

Number at risk:	CR+	19	14	10	6	3	1
	CR−	22	16	11	6	3	1

FIGURE 5 Event-free survival in surgically treated patients with (CR+) and without (CR−) contractile reserve. *Source*: From Ref. 24.

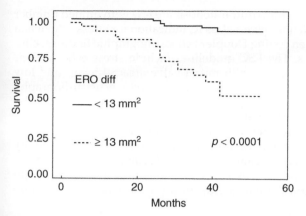

FIGURE 6 Survival curves according to changes in the severity of mitral regurgitation during exercise. *Abbreviations*: diff, difference exercise vs. rest; ERO, effective regurgitant orifice. *Source:* From Ref. 27.

severe asymptomatic mitral regurgitation that develop pulmonary hypertension with exercise (>60 mm Hg) may be considered for surgery (ACC/AHA class IIa indication). The ESC guidelines do not include stress test as part of the routine evaluation.

In patients with ischemic mitral regurgitation, stress test is useful for detecting residual myocardial ischemia, worsening mitral regurgitation (dynamic mitral regurgitation), and estimation of pulmonary artery pressures. Grading changes in mitral regurgitation severity with exercise is technically challenging and may be better accomplished with bicycle ergometry. Lancellotti et al. (27–29) have extensively studied patient with ischemic mitral regurgitation. Their protocol (30) consists in performing symptom limited, graded, semi-supine bicycle exercise with continuous two-dimensional and Doppler echocardiographic interrogation. The initial workload is 25 W for 6 minutes, with 25-W increments every 2 minutes. The severity of mitral regurgitation is estimated quantitatively (PISA) and semiquantitavely (vena contracta, jet area). They were able to prove that quantification of mitral regurgitation is possible during stress test and that there is a significant dynamic component in the severity of regurgitation in these patients. In addition, in patients with ischemic left ventricular dysfunction, large increases in mitral regurgitation during stress echo appear to identify patients at high risk of morbidity and mortality (Fig. 6).

B. Mitral Stenosis

Echocardiography is the main imaging modality for diagnosing the presence and severity of rheumatic mitral stenosis. Indication for intervention in these patients is usually based on progressive symptoms, development of atrial fibrillation and pulmonary hypertension. It is sometimes difficult to evaluate symptoms when these occurred gradually and the patient has curtailed physical activities to avoid them (loops 72a–b). On the other hand, there are patients with moderate degree of mitral stenosis but disabling symptoms. In both circumstance, stress echocardiography is an invaluable technique for the comprehensive evaluation of these patients.

The studies using stress echo in mitral stenosis are few with limited number of patients. ACC/AHA guidelines give a class IC indication for stress echo when there is a discrepancy between resting Doppler echocardiographic findings, clinical findings, and symptoms. The ESC guidelines include stress echo in their flowchart for asymptomatic patients with mitral valve area >1.5 cm^2 and low risk of embolism or hemodynamic decompensation. Exercise echocardiography is the preferred technique to evaluate these patients (31–34). Dobutamine echo has also been reported in patients unable to exercise (35,36), but is not routinely used. Mitral valve gradients pre- and postexercise as well as tricuspid jet velocity for estimation of pulmonary hypertension should be obtained (loops 73a–b). Development of severe mitral regurgitation with exercise in patients with mitral stenosis has been reported and may explain symptoms in some patients with milder degree of mitral regurgitation (37,38). In my experience this is a rare occurrence.

III. PERSONAL PERSPECTIVE

Stress echo is an essential tool in the evaluation of patients with valvular heart disease. Although it is recognized that it is underutilized, the lack of large prospective validation studies has undermine its role in clinical practice. The recent guidelines of the American Society of Echocardiography (3) on application of stress echocardiography briefly mention the indication of valvular heart disease. In our institution, this technique has a prominent role in assessing symptoms and hemodynamic significance of valvular lesions. We have to be aware of the indications, limitations, and safety issues of stress echo in this setting. In addition, to obtain meaningful data it is crucial to have necessary skills to interpret Doppler hemodynamics and apply quantitative methods for stenotic and regurgitant lesions.

DVD note: The following loops are related to the content of this chapter: 70a–b, 71a–c, 72a–b, 73a–b. These loops can be found in the provided DVD.

REFERENCES

1. Bonow RO, Carabello BA, Kanu C, et al. ACC/AHA 2006 guidelines for the management of patients with valvular heart disease: A report of the American College of Cardiology/American Heart Association Task Force on Practice Guidelines (writing committee to revise the 1998 Guidelines for the Management of Patients with Valvular Heart Disease): Developed in collaboration with the Society of Cardiovascular Anesthesiologists: Endorsed by the Society for Cardiovascular Angiography and Interventions and the Society of Thoracic Surgeons. Circulation 2006; 114(5):e84–e231.
2. Vahanian A, Baumgartner H, Bax J, et al. Guidelines on the management of valvular heart disease: The Task Force on the Management of Valvular Heart Disease of the European Society of Cardiology. Eur Heart J 2007; 28(2):230–268.
3. Pellikka PA, Nagueh SF, Elhendy AA, et al. American Society of Echocardiography recommendations for performance, interpretation, and application of stress echocardiography. J Am Soc Echocardiogr 2007; 20(9):1021–1041.
4. Otto CM, Burwash IG, Legget ME, et al. Prospective study of asymptomatic valvular aortic stenosis. Clinical, echocardiographic, and exercise predictors of outcome. Circulation 1997; 95(9):2262–2270.
5. Amato MC, Moffa PJ, Werner KE, et al. Treatment decision in asymptomatic aortic valve stenosis: Role of exercise testing. Heart 2001; 86(4):381–386.

6. Lancellotti P, Lebois F, Simon M, et al. Prognostic importance of quantitative exercise Doppler echocardiography in asymptomatic valvular aortic stenosis. Circulation 2005; 112(9 suppl):I377–I382.
7. Das P, Rimington H, Chambers J. Exercise testing to stratify risk in aortic stenosis. Eur Heart J 2005; 26(13):1309–1313.
8. Bermejo J, Yotti R. Low-gradient aortic valve stenosis: Value and limitations of dobutamine stress testing. Heart 2007; 93(3):298–302.
9. Bountioukos M, Kertai MD, Schinkel AF, et al. Safety of dobutamine stress echocardiography in patients with aortic stenosis. J Heart Valve Dis 2003; 12(4):441–446.
10. deFilippi CR, Willett DL, Brickner ME, et al. Usefulness of dobutamine echocardiography in distinguishing severe from nonsevere valvular aortic stenosis in patients with depressed left ventricular function and low transvalvular gradients. Am J Cardiol 1995; 75(2):191–194.
11. Grayburn PA. Assessment of low-gradient aortic stenosis with dobutamine. Circulation 2006; 113(5):604–606.
12. Lange RA, Hillis LD. Dobutamine stress echocardiography in patients with low-gradient aortic stenosis. Circulation 2006; 113(14):1718–1720.
13. Monin JL, Gueret P. Dobutamine hemodynamics for aortic stenosis with left ventricular dysfunction. Ann Cardiol Angeiol (Paris) 2005; 54(3):107–111.
14. Monin JL, Monchi M, Gest V, et al. Aortic stenosis with severe left ventricular dysfunction and low transvalvular pressure gradients: Risk stratification by low-dose dobutamine echocardiography. J Am Coll Cardiol 2001; 37(8):2101–2107.
15. Monin JL, Monchi M, Gest V, et al. Low-gradient aortic stenosis: Operative risk stratification and predictors for long-term outcome: A multicenter study using dobutamine stress hemodynamics. Circulation 2003; 108(3):319–324.
16. Schwammenthal E, Vered Z, Moshkowitz Y, et al. Dobutamine echocardiography in patients with aortic stenosis and left ventricular dysfunction: Predicting outcome as a function of management strategy. Chest 2001; 119(6):1766–1777.
17. Zuppiroli A, Mori F, Olivotto I, et al. Therapeutic implications of contractile reserve elicited by dobutamine echocardiography in symptomatic, low-gradient aortic stenosis. Ital Heart J 2003; 4(4):264–270.
18. Monin JL, Monchi M, Kirsch ME, et al. Low-gradient aortic stenosis: Impact of prosthesis-patient mismatch on survival. Eur Heart J 2007; 28(21):2620–2626.
19. Quere JP, Monin JL, Levy F, et al. Influence of preoperative left ventricular contractile reserve on postoperative ejection fraction in low-gradient aortic stenosis. Circulation 2006; 113(14):1738–1744.
20. Wahi S, Marwick TH. Aortic regurgitation reduces the accuracy of exercise echocardiography for diagnosis of coronary artery disease. J Am Soc Echocardiogr 1999; 12(11):967–973.
21. Wahi S, Haluska B, Pasquet A, et al. Exercise echocardiography predicts development of left ventricular dysfunction in medically and surgically treated patients with asymptomatic severe aortic regurgitation. Heart 2000; 84(6):606–614.
22. Percy RF, Miller AB, Conetta DA. Usefulness of left ventricular wall stress at rest and after exercise for outcome prediction in asymptomatic aortic regurgitation. Am Heart J 1993; 125(1):151–155.
23. Leung DY, Griffin BP, Stewart WJ, et al. Left ventricular function after valve repair for chronic mitral regurgitation: Predictive value of preoperative assessment of contractile reserve by exercise echocardiography. J Am Coll Cardiol 1996; 28(5):1198–1205.
24. Lee R, Haluska B, Leung DY, et al. Functional and prognostic implications of left ventricular contractile reserve in patients with asymptomatic severe mitral regurgitation. Heart 2005; 91(11):1407–1412.
25. Haluska BA, Short L, Marwick TH. Relationship of ventricular longitudinal function to contractile reserve in patients with mitral regurgitation. Am Heart J 2003; 146(1):183–188.
26. Lee R, Hanekom L, Marwick TH, et al. Prediction of subclinical left ventricular dysfunction with strain rate imaging in patients with asymptomatic severe mitral regurgitation. Am J Cardiol 2004; 94(10):1333–1337.

27. Lancellotti P, Gerard PL, Pierard LA. Long-term outcome of patients with heart failure and dynamic functional mitral regurgitation. Eur Heart J 2005; 26(15):1528–1532.
28. Lancellotti P, Lebrun F, Pierard LA. Determinants of exercise-induced changes in mitral regurgitation in patients with coronary artery disease and left ventricular dysfunction. J Am Coll Cardiol 2003; 42(11):1921–1928.
29. Lancellotti P, Troisfontaines P, Toussaint AC, et al. Prognostic importance of exercise-induced changes in mitral regurgitation in patients with chronic ischemic left ventricular dysfunction. Circulation 2003; 108(14):1713–1717.
30. Lebrun F, Lancellotti P, Pierard LA. Quantitation of functional mitral regurgitation during bicycle exercise in patients with heart failure. J Am Coll Cardiol 2001; 38(6):1685–1692.
31. Lev EI, Sagie A, Vaturi M, et al. Value of exercise echocardiography in rheumatic mitral stenosis with and without significant mitral regurgitation. Am J Cardiol 2004; 93(8):1060–1063.
32. Tunick PA, Freedberg RS, Gargiulo A, et al. Exercise Doppler echocardiography as an aid to clinical decision making in mitral valve disease. J Am Soc Echocardiogr 1992; 5(3):225–230.
33. Aviles RJ, Nishimura RA, Pellikka PA, et al. Utility of stress Doppler echocardiography in patients undergoing percutaneous mitral balloon valvotomy. J Am Soc Echocardiogr 2001; 14(7):676–681.
34. Schwammenthal E, Vered Z, Agranat O, et al. Impact of atrioventricular compliance on pulmonary artery pressure in mitral stenosis: An exercise echocardiographic study. Circulation 2000; 102(19):2378–2384.
35. Reis G, Motta MS, Barbosa MM, et al. Dobutamine stress echocardiography for noninvasive assessment and risk stratification of patients with rheumatic mitral stenosis. J Am Coll Cardiol 2004; 43(3):393–401.
36. Hecker SL, Zabalgoitia M, Ashline P, et al. Comparison of exercise and dobutamine stress echocardiography in assessing mitral stenosis. Am J Cardiol 1997; 80(10):1374–1377.
37. Tischler MD, Battle RW, Saha M, et al. Observations suggesting a high incidence of exercise-induced severe mitral regurgitation in patients with mild rheumatic mitral valve disease at rest. J Am Coll Cardiol 1995; 25(1):128–133.
38. Tischler MD, Niggel J. Exercise echocardiography in combined mild mitral valve stenosis and regurgitation. Echocardiography 1993; 10(5):453–457.

10 Stress-Echocardiography in Idiopathic Dilated Cardiomyopathy

Aleksandar N. Neskovic

Department of Cardiology, Clinical-Hospital Center Zemun, Belgrade University School of Medicine, Belgrade, Serbia

Approximately 36/100,000 persons per year in the United States are diagnosed to have idiopathic dilated cardiomyopathy (DCM), which is responsible for more than 10,000 deaths per year (1).

Choosing optimal therapeutic strategy for patients with DCM is directed mainly by present clinical status and prognostic assessment. Although it is well known that resting systolic function in these patients weakly correlates with symptoms, exercise capacity, and prognosis, and despite the fact that resting parameters do not always reflect the true severity of the disease, stress echocardiography is infrequently used in this patient population as compared to patients with coronary artery disease.

On the other hand, there are convincing evidence that stress echocardiography can be used for collecting valuable, clinically relevant information that might improve management of patients with DCM and utilization of health resources.

I. RATIONAL FOR THE USE OF STRESS ECHOCARDIOGRAPHY IN PATIENTS WITH DILATED CARDIOMYOPATHY

Peak oxygen consumption during exercise is widely considered as the most important prognostic parameter in DCM patients (2). However, it is not determined exclusively by cardiovascular factors and various parameters may influence maximal oxygen consumption during cardiopulmonary testing and test interpretation (i.e., age, sex, muscle mass, regular physical exercise, skeletal muscle dysfunction) (3–5). In fact, DCM patients with different severity of cardiovascular impairment may reveal similar maximal oxygen consumption, and more data are needed for precise risk stratification (6).

The use of stress echocardiography in patients with DCM is based on the concept of contractile reserve. It has been shown that assessment of contractile reserve by stress echocardiography may refine prognosis in patients with left ventricular systolic dysfunction (7–9). In particular, these studies revealed that improvement in left ventricular function, maximal oxygen consumption, and survival during follow-up can be predicted by the magnitude of left ventricular myocardium contractile response to inotropic stimulation.

This response can be measured by stress-induced changes in ejection fraction, left ventricular volumes, wall motion score index, or the rate of left ventricular pressure rise.

Gradual changes in resting left ventricular function and stress-induced functional changes (Fig. 1) can be detected during the progression of the

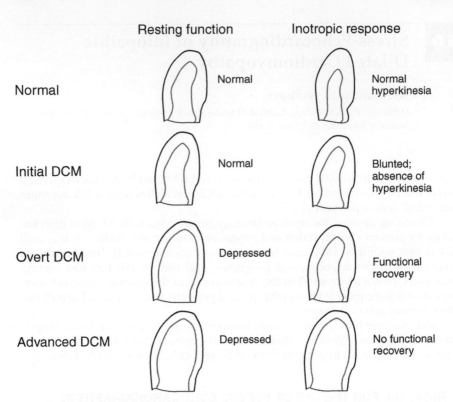

Resting function   Inotropic response

Normal   Normal   Normal
                                                    hyperkinesia

Initial DCM   Normal   Blunted;
                                                    absence of
                                                    hyperkinesia

Overt DCM   Depressed   Functional
                                                    recovery

Advanced DCM   Depressed   No functional
                                                    recovery

FIGURE 1 Resting left ventricular function and reponse to inotropic stimulation in normal individuals and in patients with various stages of idiopathic dilated cardiomyopathy. *Abbreviation*: DCM, idiopathic dilated cardiomyopathy.

myocardial disease in DCM patients (10). Normal response to inotropic stimulation is increase in contractility (hypercontractility) as compared to resting (baseline) function. In early stage of myocardial disease, myocardial function impairment may be too subtle to influence resting myocardial function, which frequently appears normal during baseline echocardiographic assessment. However, during inotropic stimulation, normally expected hypercontractility response could be absent or blunted. Progression of the disease can be verified during follow-up by gradual decrease of resting left ventricular function, characteristically associated with reduction or absence of contractile response to inotropic stimulation. Finally, poor resting left ventricular function and no response to inotropic stimulation indicate advanced disease and dismal prognosis. Importantly, the rate of deterioration of left ventricular function is influenced by the nature of the disease with wide variations in individual patients and may favorably be altered by appropriate and timely therapeutic interventions.

II. STRESS ECHOCARDIOGRAPHY PROTOCOLS IN PATIENTS WITH DILATED CARDIOMYOPATHY

In contrast to ischemia and viability testing, stress echocardiography in patients with DCM is not widely offered as routine test procedure in echocardiographic laboratories. Thus, currently it is underused, mainly due to lack of expertise and experience with the technique in this clinical setting and the absence of general consensus about the optimal protocol for assessing contractile reserve in patients with left ventricular systolic dysfunction.

A. Stress Protocols

The main goal is to quantify left ventricular contractile reserve, defined as the difference between the value of the measured index of contractility at peak inotropic stimulation and the resting (baseline) values.

Different stressors can be used for this purpose: dobutamine, dipyridamole, or exercise.

Dobutamine Stress Echocardiography

Most authors withdraw β-blockers prior to stress echocardiography, but some do not. Either low- or high-dose dobutamine echocardiography protocols can be used (11,12). Low-dose is usually defined as 10 μg/kg/min of dobutamine (11), although some authors also consider 20 μg/kg/min as a low-dose infusion (13). High-dose is uniformly defined as 40 μg/kg/min (7). Also, there is no consensus on the duration of each stage of dobutamine infusion—some authors use 3-minute stage (14), while the others use 5-minute stage (7). Atropine is generally not used to achieve submaximal heart rate.

We believe that the use of high-dose dobutamine and longer duration of each stage of dobutamine infusion (5 minutes instead of 3 minutes) may be helpful to evoke full contractile reserve. Altered left ventricular geometry and significant β-receptor downregulation that are typically present in DCM, may impede recruitment of full-contractile potential and these patients may show no response to low-dose dobutamine infusion despite actual presence of contractile reserve.

Importantly, the use of high-dose dobutamine is not associated with serious complications in DCM patients and it is feasible in nearly 90% of cases. The most common reason for stopping of dobutamine infusion is the occurrence of complex ventricular arrhythmias (frequent multifocal ventricular extrasystoles in 6.4% and nonsustained ventricular tachycardia in 1.6%) (7). Routine serum potassium level check prior to high-dose dobutamine stress echocardiography testing might be considered to avoid potassium depletion during the test (due to regular diuretic therapy) that may facilitate occurrence of complex arrhythmias. Significant hypotension (>30 mm Hg systolic blood pressure drop) is rare and, in our experience, occurs in less than 1% of cases.

Dipyridamole Stress Echocardiography

Standard high-dose dipyridamole protocol (0.84 mg over 10 minutes) can be used for the assessment of contractile reserve and risk stratification in patients with DCM (15). Capability of dipyridamole infusion to recruit myocardial inotropic reserve may be explained by complex mechanism that involves its hemodynamic, neurohormonal, and cardioprotective effects (16).

Exercise

The usual protocol for the assessment of left ventricular contractile reserve is performed on supine bicycle in incremental stages of 25 W, lasting 3 minutes each, but measured by radionuclide angiography (17) or by hemodynamic parameters (9). No data exist on the value of exercise stress echocardiography in DCM patients. However, it might be assumed that exercise stress echocardiography would have similar limitations as cardiopulmonary testing.

B. Left Ventricular Contractility Indices

All studies on stress echocardiography in DCM measured contractile reserve of the left ventricular. Although, ejection fraction and wall motion score index are the most frequently utilized, again, there is no consensus on what contractility index to use.

It is generally accepted that ≥5% increase in ejection fraction or ≥20% change from baseline ejection fraction during stress echocardiography identifies patients with preserved left ventricular contractile reserve and better prognosis (loops 74 and 75). Ejection fraction should be calculated by Simpson biplane formula.

However, ejection fraction may not accurately reflect left ventricular contractility, as it is significantly dependent on loading conditions (18). Changes in loading conditions in patients with DCM related to frequently present mitral regurgitation (higher preload, lower afterload) can lead to overestimation of true left ventricular contractility (19). Increased afterload due to activation of neuroendocrine compensatory mechanisms may cause decrease of ejection fraction (20). Exaggerated interventricular interaction in cases of DCM associated with pulmonary hypertension may also substantially alter left ventricular preload (21). Finally, dobutamine itself has variable influence on afterload; it may be associated with 5% increase or 10% decrease of afterload in patients with severe or mild heart failure, respectively (22).

Wall motion score index as traditional index for the detection of coronary artery disease, assessed by stress echocardiography, was also used as an index of left ventricular contractility to assess prognosis and functional recovery of DCM patients (7,13). Wall motion score index was determined in a standard manner, using 16-segment model. Of note, this index is semiquantitive, and inter- and intraobserver variability may be significant in DCM patients due to preexisting wall motion abnormalities and substantial number of patients with left bundle branch block. We observed substantial regional heterogeneity in response to dobutamine (Fig. 2), with mid-lateral segments showing largest variations in WMSi during dobutamine stimulation (23). Few other left ventricular contractile indices have been used for the assessment of left ventricular contractile reserve (i.e., cardiac power output, end-systolic pressure volume/ratio); however, their value for this purpose was found to be quite limited (24).

C. Right Ventricular Contractile Reserve

Right ventricular contractile reserve can be measured as the difference between right ventricular fractional area obtained at peak dobutamine dose during the test and the baseline values. Right ventricular area change >9% during the test might be considered as preserved right ventricular contractile reserve (25) (loop 76).

III. RESULTS OF SELECTED STUDIES

Potential of stress echocardiography to predict outcome in patients with idiopathic DCM was observed in numerous studies.

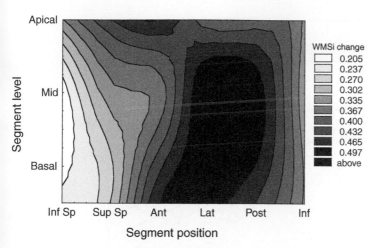

FIGURE 2 (*See color insert*) Segmental variations of wall motion score index during dobutamin stress echocardiography in patients with idiopathic dilated cardiomyopathy. Regional heterogeneity in response to dobutamine infusion with mid-lateral segments showing largest variations in wall motion score index can be noted. *Abbreviation*: WMSi, wall motion score index. *Source*: From Ref. 23.

It has been shown that changes in left ventricular wall motion score index and ejection fraction during low-dose dobutamine echocardiography are predictive of improvement of left ventricular systolic performance during medium term follow-up (13).

Preserved contractile reserve, documented by the left ventricular end-systolic volume lesser than 150 mL after dobutamine infusion and decrease of left ventricular end-diastolic volume, was associated with lower incidence off cardiac deaths or need for cardiac transplantation during long-term follow-up (26).

Peak oxygen consumption showed good correlation with contractile reserve (Fig. 3), revealing similar accuracy for predicting cardiac death or hospitalization for worsening heart failure during follow-up (14). Additionally, low-dose dobutamine may further refine prognosis in patients with "borderline" maximal oxygen consumption (between 10 and 14 mL/kg/min), since documented increase of left ventricular end-systolic diameter and systolic wall stress during inotropic stimulation with dobutamine indicates poor survival and identifies cardiac transplantation candidates (11).

Patients with atrial fibrillation–induced DCM, who show inotropic response to low-dose dobutamine, have fair chances to improve left ventricular function following restoration of sinus rhythm, in contrast with those without response, suggesting true idiopathic DCM, unlikely to show improvement during follow-up (27).

In early stages of DCM, the presence of left ventricular hypertrophy was associated with preserved myocardial contractile reserve, and late spontaneous recovery of left ventricular systolic function might be predicted by changes in left ventricular contractility and geometry induced with high-dose dobutamine (12).

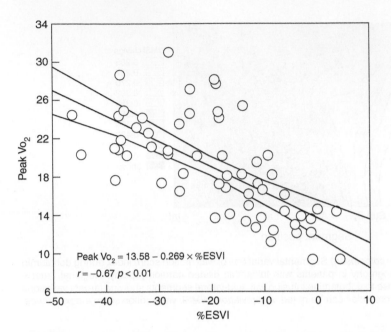

FIGURE 3 Linear correlation between peak oxygen consumption and percent change in end-systolic volume index. *Abbreviations*: %ESVI, percent change in end-systolic volume index; peak Vo₂, peak oxygen consumption. *Source*: From Ref. 14.

In the largest study to date, dobutamine-induced change in wall motion score index in 186 patients identified those at higher risk for cardiac death during the follow-up (7). Importantly, wall motion score index change was found to carry better prognostic information than change in ejection fraction, and patients with dobutamine-induced change in wall motion score index ≥0.44 are likely to have favorable prognosis (Fig. 4) (7).

We have recently shown that contractile reserve indices assessed by high-dose dobutamine correlate with myocardial histomorphometric features (24). Contractile reserve most likely reflects both the amount and the quality of contracting myocardium. Interstitial fibrosis should be inversely related to the amount of contracting myocardium, while myocyte diameter should be a robust measure of its quality. We found that myocyte diameter and interstitial fibrosis showed better correlation with change in wall motion score index than with ejection fraction. Importantly, contractile reserve indices were not equally related to the myocardial histology, since myocyte diameter consistently demonstrated stronger correlation with contractile reserve indices than interstitial fibrosis (Fig. 5) (24). Thus, it seems that the quality of contracting myocardium has more important role in dobutamine-induced contractile response than its amount.

Dipyridamole may be used to evoke contractile response instead of dobutamine, because it is less arrythmogenic (28), better tolerated, and not affected by the use of β-blocking agents, which are frequently administered in DCM patients. Recently reported overall feasibility of 99.2% for the dipyridamole stress echocardiography in prediction of prognosis in DCM patients was significantly higher as compared to previously reported feasibility of

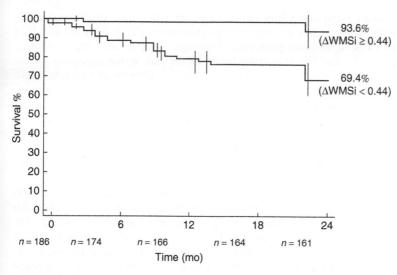

FIGURE 4 Kaplan-Meier survival curves in patients stratified according to the dobutamine-induced change in wall motion score index. Only cardiac deaths were considered. *Abbreviation*: ΔWMSi, change in wall motion score index. *Source*: From Ref. 7.

dobutamine stress echocardiography (15). Increase in wall motion score index ≥0.15 during dipyridamole stress identified patients who were more likely to survive during the mean follow-up of more than 3 years (15). In addition, combination of restrictive transmitral flow pattern (indicating severe diastolic dysfunction) and the absence of contractile response to dipyridamole was found to be particularly ominous sign, clearly associated with unfavorable outcome in patients with DCM (15).

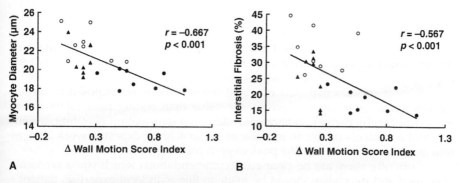

FIGURE 5 Correlation between dobutamine-induced changes in wall motion score index and myocyte diameter. Myocyte diameter (**A**) demonstrated a stronger association with dobutamine-induced changes in wall motion score index ($r = -0.67$, $p < 0.001$) than interstitial fibrosis (**B**) ($r = -0.57$, $p = 0.04$). (*Full circles*) mild histomorphometric changes, (*triangles*) moderate histomorphometric changes, and (*circles*) severe histomorphometric changes. *Abbreviation*: WMSi, wall motion score index. *Source*: From Ref. 24.

Recent study comparing head-to-head prognostic value of dipyridamole and dobutamine stress echocardiography in patients with DCM, revealed that patients with DCM who have preserved inotropic reserve after dipyridamole or dobutamine infusion are at substantially lower risk when compared with patients without inotropic reserve and that prognostic powers of two tests were similar (Fig. 6) (16). This finding may have important practical consequences, since availability of multiple pharmacologic stressors may permit the most appropriate stress to be tailored to individual patient. In this way, we can achieve flexible and versatile approach that allows choosing the test that will achieve maximal response in a given patient, taking into account possible contraindications to one test or expected limitation to interpret results of another (i.e., dobutamine stress echo in patient with ongoing β-blocker therapy).

Right ventricular contractile reserve. The impact of right ventricular function on global cardiac performance appears to be more important in patients with depressed left ventricular function as compared to normal individuals (29,30). Although it is well known that large poorly contractile right ventricle is associated with grim prognosis in patients with DCM (31,32), data are scarce on prognostic value of stress-induced changes of right ventricular performance. Increase in right ventricular ejection fraction to >35% during exercise was the only independent predictor of event-free survival in patients with advanced heart failure in one study (33), and preserved right ventricular contractile reserve (measured by pressure–area relationship) induced by low-dose dobutamine infusion was associated with a good 30-day outcome in patients with heart failure in NYHA class IV in the other study (34).

Data from our laboratory revealed limited prognostic significance of high-dose dobutamine induced change in right ventricular fractional area in patients with DCM (Fig. 7) (25). It appears that in patients with poor left ventricular contractile reserve, preserved right ventricular contractile reserve (defined as right ventricular area change of >9%) has no significant additional prognostic value, indicating crucial impact of left ventricular function on prognosis in DCM [Fig. 7(D)]. Of note, patients in whom contractile reserve of both ventricles is preserved are likely to have best prognosis [Fig. 7(C)].

IV. CONCLUDING REMARKS

Stress echocardiography should be offered for the prognostic assessment in patients with DCM especially in centers without access to cardiopulmonary testing (35).

Since it appears that data obtained when patients are exposed to certain form of stress have superior prognostic value than resting parameters, stress echocardiography may provide crucial additional information to optimize management in patients unable to exercise or fail to achieve expected work load, as well as in those with borderline peak oxygen consumption.

Currently, there are no clear-cut recommendations which stress protocols to be used and the choice should be made in line with local expertise, patient's characteristics, and preferences of attending physician.

Possible additional value of quantitative assessment of regional and global contractility during stress using novel echocardiographic techniques, like strain-rate imaging, should be clarified in future studies.

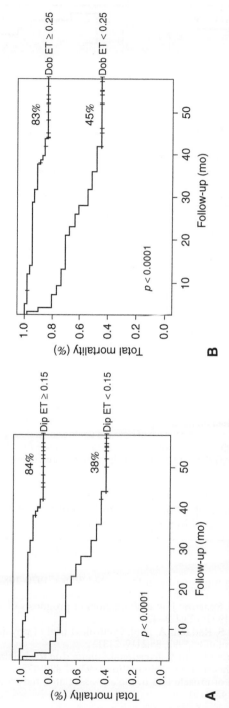

FIGURE 6 Kaplan-Meier survival curves (considering total mortality): head-to-head comparison of dipyridamole and dobutamine stress echocardiography. **(A)** Dipyridamole stress echocardiography: patients with little or no contractile response after dipyridamole infusion (Dip ET < 0.15), here identified as ΔWMSi < 0.15, showed significantly worse outcome than those with contractile reserve (Dip ET≥ 0.15). **(B)** Dobutamine stress echocardiography: patients with little or no contractile response after dobutamine infusion (Dob ET < 0.25), here identified as ΔWMSi < 0.25, showed significantly worse outcome than those with contractile reserve (Dob ET ≥ 0.25). *Source:* From Ref. 16.

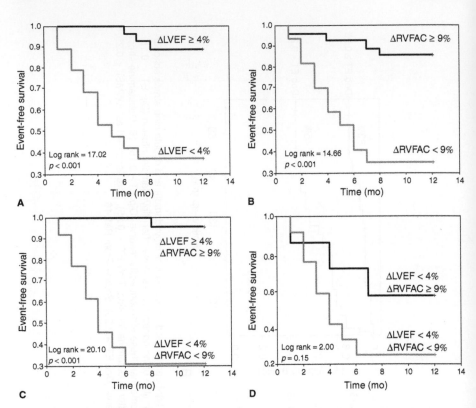

FIGURE 7 Kaplan-Meier curves for 1-year event-free survival in patients with dilated cardiomyopathy according to right and left ventricular contractile reserve and their combination. (**A**) According to LV contractile reserve, (**B**) according to RV contractile reserve, (**C**) according to either preserved or diminished contractile reserve of both the ventricles, and (**D**) according to RV contractile reserve in patients with poor LV contractile reserve. *Abbreviations*: ΔLVEF, change in left ventricular ejection fraction; ΔRVFAC, right ventricular fractional area change. *Source*: From Ref. 25.

DVD note: The following loops are related to the content of this chapter: 74–76. These loops can be found in the provided DVD.

REFERENCES

1. Gillum RF. Idiopathic cardiomyopathy in the United States, 1970–1982. Am Heart J 1986; 111:752–755.
2. Parameshwar J, Keegan J, Sparrow J, et al. Predictors of prognosis in severe chronic heart failure. Am Heart J 1992; 123:421–426.
3. Coats AJS, Adamopoulos S, Radaelli A, et al. Controlled trial of physical training in chronic heart failure. Circulation 1992; 85:2119–2131.
4. Wilson JR, Mancini DM, Dunkman B. Exertional fatigue due to skeletal muscle dysfunction in patients with heart failure. Circulation 1993; 87:470–475.
5. Fleg JL, Lakatta EG. Role of muscle loss in the age-associated reduction in $Vo_{2, max}$. J Appl Physiol 1988; 65:1147–1151.

6. Wilson JR, Rayos G, Yeoh T, et al. Dissociation between peak exercise consumption and hemodynamic dysfunction in potential heart transplant candidates. J Am Coll Cardiol 1995; 26:429–435.

7. Pratali L, Picano E, Otašević P, et al. Prognostic significance of the dobutamine echocardiography test in idiopathic dilated cardiomyopathy. Am J Cardiol 2001; 88:1374–1378.

8. Mannor A, Shneeweiss A. Prognostic value of noninvasively obtained left ventricular contractile reserve in patients with severe heart failure. J Am Coll Cardiol 1997; 29:422–428.

9. Griffin BP, Shah PK, Ferguson J, et al. Incremental prognostic value of exercise hemodynamic variables in chronic congestive heart failure secondary to coronary artery disease or to dilated cardiomyopathy. Am J Cardiol 1991; 67:848–853.

10. Picano E, Nešković A, Pratali L. Stress echocardiography in dilated cardiomyopathy. In: Picano E, ed. Stress Echocardiography, 4th ed. Berlin, Heidelberg, New York: Springer-Verlag, 2003:369–376.

11. Paraskevidis IA, Adamopoulos S, Kremastinos Th. Dobutamine echocardiographic study in patients with nonischemic dilated catdiomyopathy and prognosticall borderline values of peak exercise oxygen consumption: 18-month follow-up study. J Am Coll Cardiol 2001; 37:1685–1691.

12. Naqvi TS, Goel RK, Forrester JS, et al. Myocardial contractile reserve on dobutamine echocardiography predicts late spontaneous improvement in cardiac function in patients with recent onset idiopathic dilated cardiomyopathy. J Am Coll Cardiol 1993; 34:1537–1544.

13. Kitaoka H, Takata T, Yabe N, et al. Low dose dobutamine stress echocardiography predicts the improvement of left ventricular systolic function in dilated cardiomyopathy. Heart 1999; 81:523–527.

14. Scrutinio D, Napoli V, Passantino A, et al. Low-dose dobutamine responsivness in idiopathic dilated cardiomiopathy: Relation to exercise capacity and clinical outcome. Eur Heart J 2000; 21:927–934.

15. Pratali L, Otasevic P, Rigo F, et al. The additive prognostic value of restrictive pattern and dipyridamole-induced contractile reserve in idiopathic dilated cardiomyopathy. Eur J Heart Fail 2005; 7:844–851.

16. Pratali L, Otasevic P, Neskovic A, et al. Prognostic value of pharmacologic stress echocardiography in patients with idiopathic dilated cardiomyopathy: A prospective, head-to-head comparison between dipyridamole and dobutamine test. J Cardiac Fail 2007; 13:836–842.

17. Nagaoka H, Isobe N, Kubota S, et al. Myocardial contractile reserve as prognostic determinant in patients with idiopathic dilated cardiomyopathy without overt heart failure. Chest 1997; 111:344–350.

18. Rankin LS, Moos S, Grossman W. Alterations in preload and ejection phase indices of left ventricular performance. Circulation 1975; 51:910–919.

19. Grossman W. Evaluation of systolic and diastolic function of the myocardium. In: Baim DS, Grossman W, eds. Cardiac Catheterization, Angiography and Intervention. Baltimore, MD: Williams & Wilkins, 1996:333–358.

20. Viquerat CE, Daly P, Swedberg K. Endogenous cateholamine levels in chronic heart failure: Relation to the severity of hemodynamic abnormalities. Am J Med 1985; 78:455–460.

21. Carrol JD, Lang RM, Neumann A, et al. The differential effects of positive inotropic and vasodilator therapy in patients with congestive cardiomyopathy. Circulation 1986; 74:815–822.

22. Borow KM, Lang RM, Neumann A, et al. Physiologic mechanisms governing hemodynamic responses to positive inotropic therapy in patients with dilated cardiomyopathy. Circulation 1988; 77:625–637.

23. Neskovic AN, Otasevic P. Stress-echocardiography in evaluation of patients with idiopathic dilated cardiomyopathy. Cardiol Int 2006; 6:118–123.

24. Otasevic P, Popovic ZB, Vasiljevic JD, et al. Relation of myocardial histomorphometric features and left ventricular contractile reserve assessed by high-dose dobutamine stress echocardiography in patients with idiopathic dilated cardiomyopathy. Eur J Heart Fail 2005; 7:49–56.

25. Otasevic P, Popovic Z, Pratali L, et al. Right versus left ventricular contractile reserve in one-year prognosis of patients with idiopathic dilated cardiomiopathy: Assessment by dobutamine stress-echocardiography. Eur J Echocardiogr 2005; 6(6):429–434.

26. Drozd J, Krzeminska-Pakula M, Plewka M, et al. Prognostic value of low-dose dobutamine echocardiography in patients with dilated cardiomyopathy. Chest 2002; 121:1216–1222.

27. Paelinck B, Vermeersch P, Stockman D, et al. Usefulness of low-dose dobutamine stress echocardiography in predicting recovery of poor left ventricular function in atrial fibrillation dilated cardiomyopathy. Am J Cardiol 1999; 83:1668–1670.

28. Picano E, Marzullo P, Gigli G, et al. Identification of viable myocardium by dipyridamole-induced improvement in regional left ventricular function assessed by echocardiography in myocardial infarction and comparison with thallium scintigraphy at rest. Am J Cardiol 1992; 70:703–710.

29. Konstam MA, Cohen SR, Salem DN, et al. Comparison of left and right ventricular end-systolic pressureevolume relations in congestive heart failure. J Am Coll Cardiol 1985; 5:1326–1334.

30. Bernard D, Alpert JS. Right ventricular function in health and disease. Curr Probl Cardiol 1987; 13:423–449.

31. Sun JP, James KB, Yang XS, et al. Comparison of mortality and progression of left ventricular dysfunction in patients withi diopathic dilated cardiomyopathy and dilated versus nondilated right ventricular cavities. Am J Cardiol 1997; 80:1583–1587.

32. Lewis JF, Webber JD, Sutton LL, et al. Discordance in degree of right and left ventricular dilatation in patients with dilated cardiomyopathy: Recognition and clinical implications. J Am Coll Cardiol 1993; 21:649–654.

33. DiSalvo TG, Mathier M, Semigran MJ, et al. Preserved right ventricular ejection fraction predicts exercise capacity and survival in advanced heart failure. J Am Coll Cardiol 1995; 25:1143–1153.

34. Gorcsan J, Murali S, Counihan PJ, et al. Right ventricular performance and contractile reserve in patients with severe heart failure: Assessment by pressure–area relations and association with outcome. Circulation 1996; 94:3190–3197.

35. Neskovic AN, Otasevic P. Stress-echocardiography in idiopathic dilated cardiomyopathy: Instructions for use. Cardiovasc Ultrasound 2005; 3(1):3.

11 Risk Stratification in Noncardiac Surgery

Anai E. Durazzo
Department of Vascular Surgery, Erasmus Medical Centre, Rotterdam, The Netherlands

Sanne E. Hoeks
Department of Anaesthesiology, Erasmus Medical Centre, Rotterdam, The Netherlands

Don Poldermans
Department of Vascular Surgery, Erasmus Medical Centre, Rotterdam, The Netherlands

I. BACKGROUND

Patients undergoing major noncardiac surgery are at significant risk of cardiovascular morbidity and mortality (1,2). It is estimated that in Europe annually 40 million surgical procedures are performed, with a postoperative myocardial infarction (PMI) rate of 1% (400,000) and a cardiovascular mortality rate of 0.3% (133,000). Although the perioperative event rate has declined over the past 30 years in consequence of recent developments in anesthesiological and surgical techniques, for example, loco-regional anesthesia and endovascular treatment modalities, perioperative cardiac complications remain a significant problem (1,2).

A pooled analysis found a 30-day incidence of cardiac events (PMI and cardiac death) of 2.5% for unselected patients over the age of 40 years (1). These complications were higher in vascular surgery patients who experienced a 6.2% event rate (2). The risk of PMI is a summation of both the patients' risk and the cardiac stress related to the surgical procedure (Fig. 1). In addition, the incidence is also related to the postoperative surveillance screening adopted, as the vast majority of cardiac events (75%) are asymptomatic (3). Studies that routinely performed postoperative cardiac isoenzymes, that is, troponin T or I measurements, detected an incidence of PMI up to 25% in high-risk patients (4,5).

Preoperative cardiac risk assessment is the cornerstone of rationale perioperative management of patients scheduled for noncardiac surgery. In general, according to the American College of Cardiology/American Heart Association guidelines, indications for preoperative testing are similar to those in the nonoperative setting, being recommended in all patients at increased cardiac risk based on clinical risk profile, functional exercise capacity, and type of surgery, in whom test results will affect patient treatment and outcomes (6). Major determinants of adverse postoperative outcome are left ventricular dysfunction, aortic valve stenosis, and coronary artery disease (CAD) (Table 1). In this chapter, we will discuss the potential use of preoperative testing modalities, taking into account the pathophysiology of PMI's and the implications of test results on management and long-term outcome.

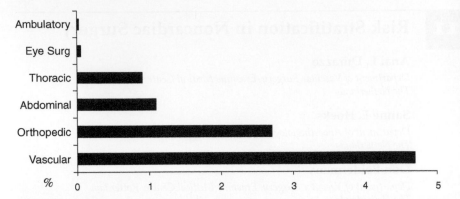

FIGURE 1 Incidence (%) of perioperative cardiac death and myocardial infarction according to the type of surgery.

II. PERIOPERATIVE MYOCARDIAL INFARCTION

Although the pathophysiology of a PMI is not entirely clear, there is evidence that coronary plaque rupture, leading to thrombus formation and subsequent vessel occlusion, is an important causative mechanism. This is similar to myocardial infarctions occurring in the nonoperative setting (7,8) (Table 2). The incidence of plaque rupture, with superimposed thrombosis, is increased by the stress response to major surgery. The perioperative surgical stress response includes a catecholamine surge with associated hemodynamic stress, vasospasm, reduced fibrinolytic activity, platelet activation, and consequent hypercoagulability (9,10). In patients with severe CAD, PMI may also be caused by a sustained myocardial supply/demand imbalance due to prolonged tachycardia and increased myocardial contractility (9–11). The association of PMI with prolonged, severe, perioperative myocardial ischemia, and the frequency of nontransmural or circumferential subendocardial infarction in the operative setting support this mechanism (9–11). Finally, hemodynamic stress and multivessel coronary disease would tend to exacerbate the extent of infarction caused by primary plaque rupture. Studies evaluating the pathophysiology of PMI using noninvasive tests, coronary angiography, and autopsy results showed that coronary plaque rupture occurred in approximately 50% of all fatal cases, while a sustained mismatch of oxygen supply and demand was responsible for the remaining (7–9,11–13). In a retrospective cohort study performed between 1989 and 2000, Poldermans et al. analyzed 32 patients who had undergone preoperative dobutamine stress

TABLE 1 The Association Between Preoperative Echocardiographic Findings and Cardiac Events in Patients Undergoing High-Risk Surgery

Perioperative cardiac events	Odds ratio (95% CI)
Myocardial ischemia	40 (5.3–292)
Left ventricular dysfunction	3.0 (1.3–6.9)
Aortic stenosis	4.8 (1.4–16)

TABLE 2 Pathophysiology of Perioperative Myocardial Infarction

---

Increased plaque rupture and thrombus formation
   Electrocardiography: ST elevation
   Inflammation plays a major role
   Therapy: aspirin, statins, and chronic β-blockers
Sustained ischemia
   Electrocardiography: ST depression
   Myocardial supply/demand mismatch
   Therapy: β-blockers and revascularization

---

echocardiography (DSE), died within 30 days of elective major vascular surgery, and had available autopsy results. Inducible ischemia on DSE was noted in 16 out of 32 patients and all 16 of these patients had PMI. However, five patients without preoperative stress-induced ischemia also exhibited evidence of recent myocardial ischemia at autopsy. The location of PMI was less accurately identified by preoperative DSE. Although the area of stress-induced ischemia corresponded with the anatomic location of infarction in 81% of the patients, in 56% of the patients the PMI extended beyond the ischemic territory (13) (Fig. 2). In a recent study of Feringa et al., 401 vascular surgery patients were evaluated by continuous 12-lead electrocardiographic monitoring during surgery and evaluated for the presence and location of ischemia in relation to the preoperative assessed coronary artery culprit lesion and inflammatory status. In addition, myocardial ischemia was divided into ST-segment depression or elevation, representing subendocardial and transmural ischemia, respectively. Myocardial

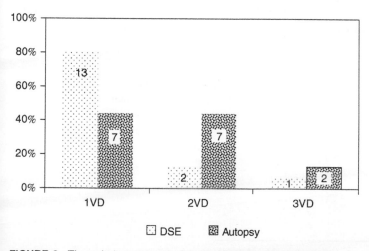

FIGURE 2 The culprit coronary lesion assessed by stress-induced wall motion abnormalities during dobutamine stress echocardiography and infarction at autopsy. The left bars represent the number of patients with myocardial ischemia during dobutamine stress echocardiography with respectively 1, 2, or 3 vessels disease. The right bars indicate the number of patients with infarction at autopsy with respectively 1, 2, or 3 vessels disease. *Abbreviations*: VD, vessel disease; DSE, dobutamine stress echocardiography. *Source*: From Ref. 13.

TABLE 3 Baseline Characteristics of 401 Patients Using Perioperative Electrocardiographic Recordings According to ST-Segment Changes

Characteristics	No change ($n = 306$)	ST- ↓ ($n = 65$)	ST- ↑ ($n = 30$)
Age (yr)	66 ± 10	71 ± 8[a]	67 ± 11
Angina pectoris	47 (15%)	17 (26%)[a]	7 (23%)[a]
Myocardial infarction	94 (31%)	32 (49%)[a]	21 (70%)[a]
High-sensitive CRP (mg/dL)	14 ± 27	53 ± 41[a]	82 ± 45[a]
Leucocytes × 10⁹ (cells/mL)	8.5 ± 2.9	8.5 ± 2.6	10 ± 2[a]
Agreement location of preoperative coronary culprit lesion and perioperative ECG changes (%)		89	53[a]

↓: Depression; ↑: elevation.
[a] *p*-value < 0.01.
Abbreviation: CRP, C-reactive protein.
Source: From Ref. 14.

ischemia was detected in 24% of the patients, ST-depression in 16%, and ST-elevation in 8%. Patients with ST-elevation had significantly higher inflammatory status when high-sensitive C-reactive protein (CRP) and leukocyte count were evaluated compared to those with ST-depression. Importantly, the preoperative assessed culprit coronary lesion location by noninvasive stress testing was related to ST-depression in 89% and ST-elevation in only 53% ($p < 0.001$) (14) (Fig. 3; Table 3). These studies showed one of the limitations of preoperative cardiac risk assessment focusing on the identification of the culprit coronary artery lesion. Using cardiac testing, one can identify the patient at risk; however, the location of the PMI is difficult to foresee due to the unpredictable progression of (asymptomatic) coronary artery lesions toward unstable plaques due to the stress of surgery in which the inflammatory status plays a major role.

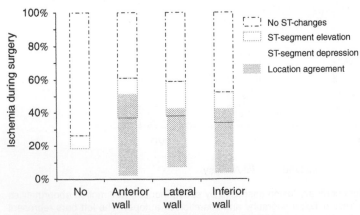

FIGURE 3 Stress-induced myocardial ischemia prior to surgery related to ST changes during high-risk surgery. *Source*: From Ref. 14.

III. AORTIC VALVE STENOSIS

Aortic valve stenosis is the most common valvular heart disease in the western society affecting 2% to 9% of adults over 65 years of age. Aortic valve stenosis is a risk factor for cardiac complications in patients undergoing noncardiac surgery (15). In a retrospective cohort study performed between 1991 and 2000, the incidence of postoperative cardiac events was increased in patients with aortic stenosis compared to those without it (14% vs. 2%, respectively). In this study, patients with aortic stenosis had an almost sevenfold increased risk of cardiac events, regardless of the presence of risk factors for CAD, such as angina, previous myocardial infarction, heart failure, renal dysfunction, and stroke (16). These findings are in agreement with prior research and guidelines based initially on the study by Goldman et al., who in 1977 reported major cardiac complications in 13% of 23 patients with important aortic stenosis (17). The pathophysiology of cardiac events is related to an interaction of developing hypotension and low cardiac output during surgery and underlying CAD. Importantly, the outcome was worse in patients with more advanced aortic valve disease. In patients with an aortic valve area <0.7 cm^2 or a mean gradient >50 mm Hg, the incidence of cardiac events was 31%, while in patients with an aortic valve area 0.7 to 1 cm^2 or a mean gradient 25 to 49 mm Hg, the incidence of cardiac events was 11% (15).

IV. LEFT VENTRICULAR DYSFUNCTION

The prognostic value of left ventricular function for perioperative cardiac events has changed over time. Initially, this was an important factor of clinical risk indexes, such as Goldman's (17) or Detsky's (18) risk score. The study of Kazmers et al. (19), evaluating left ventricular function as dichotomous variable prior to vascular surgery in 1988, found a cutoff of 35% as optimal predictor of postoperative cardiac events. However, the recently introduced assessment of myocardial viability during stress testing has changed the impact of left ventricular dysfunction. As shown in a study of 295 patients with a left ventricular ejection fraction <35% scheduled for vascular surgery, postoperative cardiac events were related to the presence of stress-induced ischemia and scar tissue, but inversely related to the presence of sustained improvement. Using multivariate analysis, the number of ischemic segments was associated with perioperative cardiac events [odds ratio per segment, 1.6; 95% confidence interval (CI), 1.05–1.8], whereas the number of segments with sustained improvement was associated with improved outcome (odds ratio per segment, 0.2; 95% CI, 0.04–0.7) (20). Although, reduced left ventricular function is a moderate preoperative cardiac risk factor, the stratification using stress testing enables the physician to identify a subgroup of patients with sustained improvement who have a relatively benign postoperative outcome, conversely to patients with a predominant ischemic response.

V. CARDIAC RISK STRATIFICATION

Adequate preoperative cardiac risk assessment is fundamental to identify patients at risk for adverse postoperative outcome. Numerous investigators have described the relationship between patient characteristics and the risk of adverse cardiovascular outcome. Based on specific clinical risk factors that allow an estimation of the weighted risk of perioperative cardiac complications, several risk indices have been developed in the past, including the Goldman cardiac risk index (17), the Detsky modified multifactorial risk index (18), and Eagle's

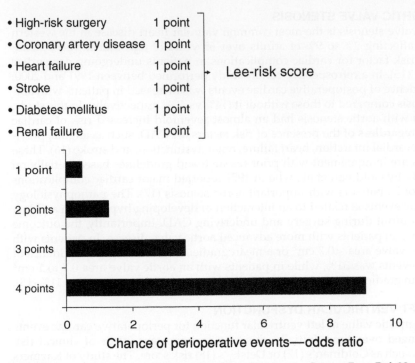

FIGURE 4   Lee risk score and chance of perioperative events. *Source*: From Ref. 23.

risk score (21). It was observed that no index was significantly superior to the other (22). However, in 1999, Lee and colleagues revised the Goldman risk index. They developed the most commonly used risk model, the Revised Cardiac Risk Index, which has a superior predictive value, compared to previous risk models (23). This "simplified index," identifies six independent predictors of major cardiac complications: (1) high-risk surgery, (2) ischemic heart disease, (3) congestive heart failure, (4) cerebrovascular disease, (5) diabetes, and (6) renal failure. Increasing numbers of risk factors correlate with an increased risk. Based on the presence of 0, 1, 2, or ≥3 risk factors, the estimated cardiac event rate was 0.4%, 0.9%, 7%, and 11%, respectively (Fig. 4). Further risk stratification could be achieved by a refinement of the risk of the surgical procedure and the addition of elderly age as a risk factor. By stratification, the type of surgery into low-, intermediate-low, intermediate-high, and high-risk surgery in a cohort of 108.593 patients, the predictive value of the Revised Cardiac Risk Index was significantly improved, compared to a dichotomous stratification of the surgical risk. (C-statistic improved from 0.63 to 0.85) (24).

The next issue is to identify those patients who should undergo additional stress testing before surgery. Based on the recently published *American College of Cardiology/American Heart Association (ACC/AHA) 2007 Guidelines on Perioperative Cardiovascular Evaluation and Care for Noncardiac Surgery* (6), and *European Society of Cardiology 2009 Guidelines for Pre-operative Cardiac Risk Assessment and Perioperative Cardiac Management in Non-cardiac Surgery* (25), the patient's clinical risk, functional status, and the surgery-specific cardiac risk are considered to determine which patients are candidates for cardiac testing.

1. Patients in need for emergency noncardiac surgery further cardiac risk assessment or treatments are usually initiated after patient has recovered from surgery.
2. Patients being considered for elective noncardiac surgery, but with an active cardiac condition defined as the presence of unstable coronary disease, decompensate heart failure, significant arrhythmias, and severe valvular disease; the surgery is usually cancelled or delayed, until the cardiac problem has been clarified and treated appropriately. Discontinuation of aspirin therapy should be considered only in those patients in which hemostasis is difficult to control during surgery (25).
3. Patients undergoing low-risk surgical procedures, many of which associated with a combined morbidity and mortality rate less than 1%, cardiovascular testing will rarely result in a change in management even in high-risk patients. Therefore, it is appropriate to proceed directly with the planned surgical procedure.
4. Functional capacity has been shown to be reliable for perioperative and long-term prediction of cardiac events (26). In highly functional asymptomatic patients, management will hardly ever be changed based on the results of any additional cardiovascular testing, being appropriate to proceed with the planned low-, intermediate-, or high-risk surgery.
5. Patients with poor or unknown functional capacity, then the presence of clinical risk factors, evaluated by the Revised Cardiac Risk Index (23), will determine the need for further evaluation.

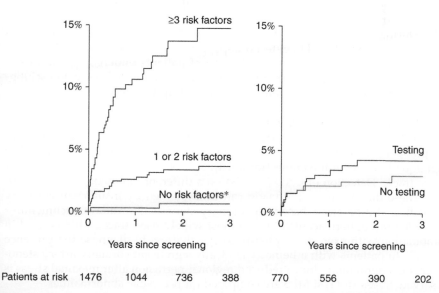

FIGURE 5 Perioperative and long-term cardiac events according to baseline risk factors. Patients with one or two risk factors were stratified for additional preoperative cardiac testing. As shown, the use of stress test results did not improve outcome.

6. If the patient has no clinical risk factors, then it is appropriate to proceed with the planned surgery.
7. If the patient with poor or unknown functional capacity has 1 or 2 clinical risk factors, then it is reasonable to either proceed with the planned surgery with tight heart rate control using β-blockade and statins, or consider testing if it will change management (Fig. 5).
8. In patients with three or more clinical risk factors undergoing intermediate-risk surgery, testing may be considered if the results will change management.
9. In patients with three or more clinical risk factors undergoing high-risk surgery, it is reasonable to perform testing if the results will change management.

VI. ASSESSMENT OF RISK FOR CORONARY ARTERY DISEASE

A. Exercise Electrocardiogram

The most commonly used physiological stress test for detecting myocardial ischemia is treadmill or cycle ergometer test. The advantages are that it provides an estimate of the functional capacity, hemodynamic response, and detects myocardial ischemia by ST-segment changes. The accuracy of the exercise ECG varies widely among studies. Meta-analysis by Kertai et al. for detection of myocardial ischemia with treadmill testing in vascular surgery patients showed a rather low sensitivity (74%; 60–88%) and specificity (69%; 60–78%), comparable to daily clinical practice (27). However, important limitations in patients with peripheral vascular disease are their frequently limited exercise capacity. Furthermore, a preexistent ST-segment deviation, especially in the precordial leads V5 and V6 on the rest ECG makes a reliable ST-segment analysis more difficult (28).

During the past decades, different noninvasive and nonphysiological stress tests have been developed to detect preoperative myocardial ischemia. The main techniques used in preoperative evaluation of patients undergoing noncardiac surgery who cannot exercise are the radionuclide myocardial perfusion scintigraphy (MPS) and dobutamine stress echocardiography (DSE).

B. Myocardial Perfusion Scintigraphy

Myocardial perfusion scintigraphy is a widely used nonexercise technique in the preoperative risk assessment of patients undergoing vascular surgery. The technique involves intravenous administration of a small quantity of a radioactive tracer. Detection of CAD is based on a difference in blood flow distribution. These differences in perfusion can be explained by insufficient coronary blood flow during stress based on coronary stenosis. Nowadays, technicum99 m-labeled radiopharmaceutical is the most widely used tracer. MPS is used in combination with exercise or pharmacological stress to diagnose the presence of CAD. In patients with a hemodynamically significant coronary artery stenosis or transmural infarction, a reduced regional perfusion after maximal stress is observed. Stress and rest MPS are compared for reversible abnormalities.

These noninvasive tests have been studied extensively. Most studies indicate that reversible perfusion defects, which reflect viable myocardium, carry the greatest risk of perioperative cardiac death or PMI, while a fixed perfusion defects predict long-term cardiac events. This technique is highly sensitive for prediction of cardiac complications but the specificity has been reported less satisfactory; studies show that the positive predictive value of reversible defects range from 2% to 20%, and the negative predictive value of a normal scan is around 99% (6).

Several studies have shown that the risk of cardiac events increases as the amount of myocardium at risk, reflected in the extent of reversible defects found in imaging. A meta-analysis by Etchells et al. (29) investigated the prognostic value of semiquantitative dipyridamole MPS for perioperative cardiac risk in patients undergoing noncardiac vascular surgery. They included nine studies involving a total of 1179 vascular surgery patients with a 7% cardiac complication rate. One of the most important findings in this study was that reversible ischemia in less than 20% of the myocardial segments did not change the likelihood of perioperative complications. However, when the reversible ischemia was observed in more than 20% of the myocardial segments, the perioperative cardiac event rates increased progressively as the extent of reversible defects increased.

C.   Stress Echocardiography

Initially, this test was developed to provide prognostic information following myocardial infarction, and recently has been adapted to preoperative cardiac risk assessment. As most patients with peripheral vascular disease are not able to exercise maximally, stress echocardiography with pharmacological stressors like dobutamine is a good alternative. Dobutamine, a synthetic cathecholamine, is a β_1-receptor agonist that exerts a strong inotropic but weak chronotropic effect on the heart. Although vasodilators (i.e., dipyridamol or adenosine) may have advantages for assessment of myocardial perfusion, dobutamine is the preferred pharmacological stressor when the test is based on assessment of regional wall motion abnormalities (30). During DSE, dobutamine is intravenously administered at a gradually increasing dose. The standard protocol for DSE starts with a dobutamine infusion at 5µg/kg/min and increasing at 3-minute intervals to 10, 20, 30, and 40 µg/kg/min. If signs and symptoms of ischemia are absent, atropine is given to patients who do not reach their age-corrected target heart rate [(220 - Age) × 0.85 in men and (200 - Age) × 0.85 in women] (30). During the infusion, contractility and heart rate increase, leading to increased myocardial oxygen demand, which results in myocardial ischemia and systolic contractile dysfunction in regions supplied by hemodynamically significantly CAD, assessed by echocardiography. Studies show that DSE can be performed safely and is well tolerated (30).

Tissue harmonic imaging is advised for stress echocardiography. This special imaging setting reduces near-field artifact, improves resolution, enhances myocardial signals, and is superior to fundamental imaging for endocardial border visualization. The improvement in endocardial visualization is further improved by the use of myocardial contrast agents. This has decreased interobserver variability and improved the sensitivity of stress echocardiography.

The value of DSE for preoperative cardiac risk evaluation has been extensively evaluated. In the series by Poldermans et al. (31), the left ventricular wall was divided into 16 segments, and wall motion in each was subjectively scored on a four-point scale: 1 = normal; 2 = hypokinetic; 3 = akinetic, and 4 = dyskinetic. The test results were considered positive when wall motion in any segment deteriorated one grade or more. For each patient, a wall motion score index (total

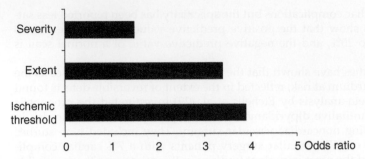

FIGURE 6 Perioperative cardiac death and nonfatal myocardial infarction chance according to the presence of dobutamine stress echocardiography abnormalities. *Source*: From Ref. 31.

score divided by the number of assessable segments) was calculated at rest and during peak stress, severity of ischemia was defined as the difference between these two values; extent of ischemia was defined as the number of segments exhibiting deterioration wall motion during stress; and ischemic threshold was defined as the heart rate at which new echocardiographic wall motion abnormalities occurred divided by the maximal age-related heart rate [(220 - Age) in men, and (200 - Age) × 0.85 in women]. The authors studied a population of 302 consecutive patients who underwent DSE before a major vascular surgery. New wall motion abnormalities occurred in 72 patients. All 27 patients with a cardiac-related event had new wall motion abnormalities during stress (negative predictive value of 100%). The positive predictive value was 38%. The presence of a new wall-motion abnormality was a powerful determinant of an increased risk for perioperative events, and the heart rate threshold at which ischemia occurred provided additional prognostic information. Patients with positive DSE test results and a low ischemic threshold (heart rate <70% of the age-corrected maximal heart rate) were at extremely high risk (Fig. 6; Table 4). Several other studies have suggested that the extent of the wall-motion abnormality and/or wall-motion change at low ischemic thresholds, particularly at a heart rate of less than 60% of age-predicted maximum, is especially important. These findings have been shown to be the predictor of long-term and short-term outcomes (31–33). The negative predictive value of DSE is high but the positive predictive value is much lower. Kertai et al. reported a weighted sensitivity of 85% (95% CI, 74–97%) and a specificity of 70% (95% CI, 62–69%) for DSE in 850 patients from 8 studies (27).

TABLE 4 Semiquantitative Analysis of Dobutamine Stress Echocardiography Test in 72 Patients with Positive Test Results According to the Presence or Absence of Perioperative Cardiac Events

	Events	No events
Threshold (heart rate)	66 (61–71)	83 (79–87)[a]
Extent (odds ratio)	3.3 (2.3–4.3)	3.6 (2.5–4.7)
Severity (odds ratio)	1.5 (1.4–1.7)	1.6 (1.4–1.8)

[a] p-value < 0.01.
Source: From Ref. 31.

D. Myocardial Perfusion Scintigraphy or Stress Echocardiography Which Test to Choose?

There is no direct comparison of these techniques in perioperative risk assessment in the same patient population. However, some meta-analyses compared the different techniques with respect to sensitivity and specificity. The recent meta-analysis by Kertai et al. on 58 studies (8119 patients) compared six different diagnostic tests for diagnostic accuracy to predict perioperative cardiac risk in patients undergoing major vascular surgery (27). There was a positive trend in favor of DSE for better diagnosis compared to other tests; however, this was only statistical significant compared to MPS. Beattie et al. conducted a meta-analysis comprising 68 studies comparing myocardium perfusion imaging versus stress echocardiography in 10.049 noncardiac surgery patients (34). The authors concluded that the likelihood ratio of a perioperative cardiac event with a positive stress echocardiography was more than twice that of a positive nuclear perfusion study (likelihood ratio, 4.09; 95% CI, 3.21–6.56 vs. likelihood ratio, 1.83; 95% CI, 1.59–2.10; and $p = 0.001$). The analysis demonstrated that a moderate-to-large perfusion defect identified by both techniques highly predicted PMI and death; however, both techniques detected only a moderate-to-large defect in 14% of the patients.

Therefore, there is no definite answer; it seems that the predictive value of MPS and DSE to assess cardiac risk in vascular patients appears to be comparable. Both tests share a very high sensitivity in detecting CAD, but both tests suffer from a lack of specificity. The choice of the test should therefore be based on the center's experience and short-term availability.

Nonetheless, DSE has some potential advantages over the other screening methods. DSE test requires shorter time to be performed than that of MPS, and can, if necessary, even be performed at the bed side; immediate availability of results; the cost is lower than that of the nuclear imaging techniques. In addition, echocardiography provides assessment not only of the global and regional functions but also valvular function. These two important conditions correlate to adverse perioperative events and imply different protective strategies to be adopted during the perioperative period. Furthermore, the heart rate that produces segmental wall motion abnormalities or electrocardiographic ST-segment depression can define an "ischemic threshold" that is potentially useful in preventing or detecting myocardial ischemia both intraoperatively and postoperatively (30,31–33,35).

However, there are also some important limitations: DSE may be nondiagnostic in patients who are on β-blocking medications, which may blunt the heart rate response; in approximately 5% of patients, the echocardiography imagining quality is insufficient for accurate analysis; and in the presence of resting regional wall motion abnormalities, the predictive accuracy for detecting ischemia is low (30,35).

VII. CONSEQUENCES CARDIAC STRESS TEST RESULTS/PERIOPERATIVE MANAGEMENT

In general, three strategies have been used in an attempt to reduce the incidence of PMIs and other cardiac complications: cancellation of surgery or perform a limited procedure, prophylactic coronary revascularization, and medical treatment.

According to the recently published American College of Cardiology/
American Heart Association (ACC/AHA) 2007 Guidelines on Perioperative
Cardiovascular Evaluation and Care for Noncardiac Surgery (6), preoperative
coronary revascularization is useful only for subgroups of high-risk patients
with unstable cardiac symptoms or those for whom coronary artery revascularization offers a long-term benefit. In the first large, randomized trial, the
Coronary Artery Revascularization Prophylaxis (CARP) trial (36), patients with
significant coronary artery stenosis schedule for vascular operations were randomly assigned to either coronary artery revascularization before surgery or
no revascularization. It was demonstrated that on the short term there is no
reduction in the number of peri- or postoperative myocardial infarctions, deaths
or length of hospital stay or in improved long-term outcome in patients who
underwent preoperative coronary revascularization compared to patients who
received optimized medical therapy. The recently randomized pilot study, the
Dutch Echocardiographic Cardiac Risk Evaluation Applying Stress Echocardiography (DECREASE) V (37) assessed the benefit of prophylactic coronary revascularization in patients with preoperative extensive stress-induced ischemia.
Patients were randomly assigned to prophylactic revascularization or optimal
medical treatment. The majority of patients had three-vessel disease. Revascularization did not improve 30 day or 1-year outcome (Fig. 7; Tables 5 and 6). These
findings of both CARP and DECREASE V trials are consistent with studies that
show that the most severe stenosis may not always be responsible for PMI and
that coronary thrombosis frequently occurs at the site of insignificant stenosis. As
a consequence, preoperative revascularization of severe stenosis may not reduce
perioperative ischemic complications. In high-risk patients scheduled for major
noncardiac vascular surgery, prophylactic revascularization might be switched
to later postoperative revascularization, preventing the delay of surgery. It has
to be noted that preoperative revascularization can even be harmful for the
patient because of periprocedural complications during revascularization and

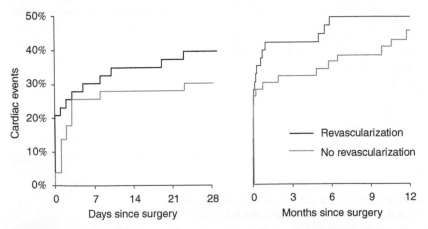

FIGURE 7 Perioperative and long-term cardiac events: the Dutch Echocardiographic Cardiac
Risk Evaluation Applying Stress Echocardiography—V study. In patients with preoperative extensive stress-induced ischemia, prophylactic revascularization did not improve 30-day or 1-year
outcome as compared to optimal medical therapy. *Source*: From Ref. 37.

TABLE 5 Preoperative Cardiac Events in Patients Undergoing High-Risk Surgery According to Preoperative Myocardial Revascularization Strategy or Not (the Dutch Echocardiographic Cardiac Risk Evaluation Applying Stress Echocardiography—V Study)

	Preoperative myocardial revascularization, N (%)	No preoperative myocardial revascularization, N (%)
Cardiovascular death	2 (4.2%)	1 (2.0%)
Myocardial infarction	1 (2.1%)	0
Composite	3 (6.3%)	1 (2.0%)

Source: From Ref. 37.

postponement of the noncardiac procedure. Importantly, the cumulative risk of prophylactic coronary revascularization and noncardiac surgery has to balance the risk of noncardiac surgery alone and the immediate benefit of prophylactic coronary revascularization.

In recent years, more attention is focused on the role of pharmacological treatment (6). Taking into consideration the pathophysiology of perioperative cardiac morbidity that mild nonobstructive lesions are also associated with MI and death, optimal medical therapy plays an importance role to prevent perioperative cardiac events. An extensive preoperative cardiac evaluation with noninvasive cardiac testing might improve the outcome by inciting an optimal medical management in the peri- and postoperative period. Perioperative β-blockers and statins have shown significant benefit in decreasing perioperative cardiac mortality and morbidity (6).

Among valvular heart disease, severe aortic stenosis poses the greatest risk for noncardiac surgery. According to the American College of Cardiology/American Heart Association (ACC/AHA) 2007 Guidelines on Perioperative Cardiovascular Evaluation and Care for Noncardiac Surgery (6), if the aortic stenosis is symptomatic, elective noncardiac surgery should be postponed or cancelled and aortic valve replacement is indicated. If the aortic stenosis is

TABLE 6 Patient Characteristics in the Dutch Echocardiographic Cardiac Risk Evaluation Applying Stress Echocardiography—II Study (DECREASE II), Coronary Artery Revascularization Prophylaxis Study (CARP), and the Dutch Echocardiographic Cardiac Risk Evaluation Applying Stress Echocardiography—V Study (DECREASE V)

Patients characteristics	DECREASE II (%)	CARP (%)	DECREASE V (%)
Angina pectoris	65	39	94
Myocardial infarction	17	42	98
Heart failure	4	10	47
Stroke	16	20	32
Diabetes	22	20	33
Renal failure	5	N/A	20

Source: From Ref. 37.

considered severe by echocardiogram analysis but asymptomatic, the surgery should be postponed or cancelled if the valve has not been evaluated within a year. In patients with severe stenosis who refuse cardiac surgery, noncardiac surgery can be performed with a mortality risk of approximately 10%. Percutaneous balloon valvuloplasty or percutaneous transcatheter valve placement may be reasonable as a bridge to surgery in those who are not candidate for surgical valve replacement, although no controlled studies are available in this setting (6,38).

VIII. CONCLUSION

The role of noninvasive tests for risk stratification in noncardiac surgery is to detect left ventricular dysfunction, aortic valve stenosis, and coronary artery disease, all major determinants of adverse postoperative outcome. Indications for preoperative risk assessment with noninvasive test, MPS and DSE, are similar to those in the nonoperative setting, being only recommended in patients at increased cardiac risk based on clinical risk profile, functional exercise capacity, and type of surgery, in whom test results will affect patient treatment and outcomes.

It seems that the predictive value of MPS or DSE for the assessment of perioperative cardiac risk appears to be comparable. Both tests share a very high sensitivity in detecting CAD, but both tests suffer from a lack of specificity. Nonetheless, DSE has some potential advantages over the other screening methods. It is an accurate, safe, cost-effective, and portable procedure for the noninvasive diagnosis of CAD. Unlike MPS, DSE offers the advantage of detecting the heart rate at which a regional wall motion abnormality occurred (ischemic threshold). In addition, echocardiography technique provides the assessment of both global and regional myocardial function, as well as valvular abnormalities.

Depending on the noninvasive tests results three strategies have been used in an attempt to reduce the incidence of PMIs and other cardiac complications: cancellation of surgery or perform a limited surgical procedure, prophylactic coronary revascularization, and optimal medical treatment.

One of the limitations of preoperative cardiac risk assessment with noninvasive tests is the identification of the culprit coronary artery lesion, as the most severe stenosis may not always be responsible for the PMI. Using cardiac testing, one can identify the patient at risk; however, the location of the perioperative myocardial infarction is difficult to foresee due to the unpredictable progression of (asymptomatic) coronary artery lesions towards unstable plaques due to the stress of surgery in which the inflammatory status plays a major role.

An extensive preoperative cardiac evaluation with noninvasive cardiac testing might improve outcome by inciting an optimal medical management in the peri- and postoperative period. Perioperative β-blockers and statins have shown significant benefit in decreasing perioperative cardiac mortality and morbidity.

REFERENCES

1. Mangano DT. Perioperative cardiac morbidity. Anesthesiology 1990; 72(1):153–184.
2. Mackey WC, Fleisher LA, Haider S, et al. Perioperative myocardial ischemic injury in high-risk vascular surgery patients: Incidence and clinical significance in a prospective clinical trial. J Vasc Surg 2006; 43(3):533–538.

3. Poldermans D, Bax JJ, Schouten O, et al. Should major vascular surgery be delayed because of preoperative cardiac testing in intermediate-risk patients receiving beta-blocker therapy with tight heart rate control? J Am Coll Cardiol 2006; 48(5): 964–969.
4. Abraham N, Lemech L, Sandroussi C, et al. A prospective study of subclinical myocardial damage in endovascular versus open repair of infrarenal abdominal aortic aneurysms. J Vasc Surg 2005; 41(3):377–380 [discussion 380–381].
5. Le Manach Y, Perel A, Coriat P, et al. Early and delayed myocardial infarction after abdominal aortic surgery. Anesthesiology 2005; 102(5):885–891.
6. Fleisher LA, Beckman JA, Brown KA, et al. ACC/AHA 2007 guidelines on perioperative cardiovascular evaluation and care for noncardiac surgery: A report of the American College of Cardiology/American Heart Association task force on practice guidelines (writing committee to revise the 2002 guidelines on perioperative cardiovascular evaluation for noncardiac surgery). J Am Coll Cardiol 2007; 50(17):e159–e241.
7. Dawood MM, Gutpa DK, Southern J, et al. Pathology of fatal perioperative myocardial infarction: Implications regarding pathophysiology and prevention. Int J Cardiol 1996; 57(1):37–44.
8. Cohen MC, Aretz TH. Histological analysis of coronary artery lesions in fatal postoperative myocardial infarction. Cardiovasc pathol 1999; 8(3):133–139.
9. Priebe HJ. Triggers of perioperative myocardial ischaemia and infarction. Br J Anaesth 2004; 93:9–20.
10. Samets W, Metzler H, Gries M, et al. Perioperative catecholamine changes in cardiac risk patients. Eur J Clin Invest 1999; 29:582–587.
11. Landesberg G. The pathophysiology of perioperative myocardial infarction: Facts and perspective. J Cardiothorac Vasc Anesth 2003; 17:90–100.
12. Ellis SG, Hertzer NR, Young JR, et al. Angiographic correlates of cardiac death and myocardial infarction complicating major nonthoracic vascular surgery. Am J Cardiol 1996; 77:1126–1128.
13. Poldermans D, Boersma E, Bax JJ, et al. Correlation of location of acute myocardial infarction after noncardiac vascular surgery with preoperative dobutamine echocardiographic findings. Am J Cardiol 2001; 88(12):1413–1414.
14. Poldermans D, Hoeks SE, Feringa HH. Pre-operative risk assessment and risk reduction before surgery. J Am Coll Cardiol 2008; 51:1913–1924.
15. Christ M, Sharkova Y, Geldner G, et al. Preoperative and perioperative care for patients with suspected or established aortic stenosis facing noncardiac surgery. Chest 2005; 128:2944–2953.
16. Kertai M, Bountioukos M, Boersma E, et al. Aortic stenosis: An underestimated risk factor for perioperative complications in patients undergoing noncardiac surgery. Am J Med 2004; 116(1):8–13.
17. Goldman L, Caldera DL, Nussbaum SR, et al. Multifactorial index of cardiac risk in noncardiac surgical procedures. N Engl J Med 1977; 297(16):845–850.
18. Detsky AS, Abrams HB, Forbath N, et al. Cardiac assessment for patients undergoing noncardiac surgery. A multifactorial clinical risk index. Arch Intern Med 1986; 146(11):2131–2134.
19. Kazmers A, Cerqueira MD, Zierler RE. Perioperative and late outcome in patients with left ventricular ejection fraction of 35% or less who require major vascular surgery. J Vasc Surg 1988; 8(3):307–315.
20. Karagiannis SE, Feringa HH, Vidakovic R, et al. Value of myocardial viability estimation using dobutamine stress echocardiography in assessing risk preoperatively before noncardiac vascular surgery in patients with left ventricular ejection fraction <35%. Am J Cardil 2007; 99(11):1555–1559.
21. Eagle KA, Coley CM, Newell JB, et al. Combining clinical and thallium data optimizes preoperative assessment of cardiac risk before major vascular surgery. Ann Intern Med 1989; 110:859–866.
22. Gilbert K, Larocque BJ, Patrick LT. Prospective evaluation of cardiac risk indices for patients undergoing noncardiac surgery. Ann Intern Med 2000; 133:356–359.

23. Lee TH, Marcantonio ER, Mangione CM, et al. Derivation and prospective validation of a simple index for prediction of cardiac risk of major noncardiac surgery. Circulation 1999; 100:1043–1049.

24. Boersma E, Kertai MD, Schouten O, et al. Perioperative cardiovascular mortality in noncardiac surgery: Validation of the Lee cardiac risk index. Am J Med 2005; 118:1134–1141.

25. Poldermans D, Bax JJ, Boersma E, et al. Guidelines for pre-operative cardiac risk assessment and perioperative cardiac management in non-cardiac surgery. The Task Force for Preoperative Cardiac Risk Assessment and Perioperative Cardiac Management in Non-cardiac Surgery of the European Society of Cardiology (ESC) and endorsed by the European Society of Anaesthesiology (ESA). European Heart Journal doi:10.1093/eurheartj/ehp337.

26. Nelson CL, Herndon JE, Mark DB, et al. Relation of clinical and angiographic factors to functional capacity as measured by Duke activity status index. Am J Cardiol 1991; 68:973–975.

27. Kertai MD, Boersma E, Bax JJ, et al. A meta-analysis comparing the prognostic accuracy of six diagnostic tests for predicting perioperative cardiac risk in patients undergoing major vascular surgery. Heart 2003; 89(11):1327–1334.

28. Gibbons RJ, Balady GJ, Timothy Bricker J, et al. ACC/AHA 2002 guideline update for exercise testing: Summary article: A report of the American College of Cardiology/American Heart Association task force on practice guidelines (committee to update the 1997 exercise testing guidelines). J Am Coll Cardiol 2002; 40(8):1531–1540.

29. Etchells E, Meade M, Tomlinson G, et al. Semiquantitative dipyridamole myocardial stress perfusion imaging for cardiac risk assessment before noncardiac vascular surgery: A meta analysis. J Vasc Surg 2002; 36(3):534–540.

30. Pellikka PA, Nagueh SF, Elhendy AA, et al. American Society of Echocardiography recommendations for performance, interpretation, and application of stress echocardiography. J Am Soc Echocardiogr 2007; 20(9):1021–1041.

31. Poldermans D, Arnese M, Fioretti PM, et al. Improved cardiac risk stratification in major vascular surgery with dobutamine-atropine stress echocardiography. J Am Coll Cardiol 1995; 26(3):648–653.

32. Poldermans D, Fioretti PM, Forster T, et al. Dobutamine stress echocardiography for assessing cardiac risk in patients having noncardiac surgery. Study of perioperative ischemia research group. Ann Intern Med 1996; 125:433–441.

33. Das MK, Pellikka PA, Mahoney DW, et al. Assessment of cardiac risk before nonvascular surgery: Dobutamine stress echocardiography in 530 patients. J Am Coll Cardiol 2000; 35:1647–1653.

34. Beattie WS, Abdelnaem E, Wijeysundera DN, et al. A meta-analytic comparison of preoperative stress echocardiography and nuclear scintigraphy imaging. Anesth Analg 2006; 102(1):8–16.

35. Pellikka PA, Roger VL, Oh JK, et al. Stress echocardiography. Part II. Dobutamine stress echocardiography: Techniques, implementation, clinical applications, and correlations. Mayo Clin Proc 1995; 70:16–27.

36. McFalls EO, Ward HB, Morits TE, et al. Coronary-artery revascularization before elective major vascular surgery. N Engl J Med 2004; 351(27):2795–2804.

37. Poldermans D, Schouten O, Vidakovic R, et al. A clinical randomized trial to evaluate the safety of a noninvasive approach in high-risk patients undergoing major vascular surgery: The DECREASE-V Pilot Study. J Am Coll Cardiol 2007; 49(17):1763–1769.

38. Cribier A, Eltchaninoff H, Bash A, et al. Percutaneous transcatheter implantation of an aortic valve prosthesis for calcific aortic stenosis: First human case description. Circulation 2002; 106:3006–3008.

Stress Echocardiography Versus Radionuclide Imaging

Georges Athanassopoulos

Onassis Cardiac Surgery Center, Athens, Greece

I. DIAGNOSIS OF CORONARY ARTERY DISEASE

Myocardial perfusion scintigraphy represents the most widely used noninvasive imaging modality for the diagnosis of coronary artery disease (CAD). The modality has high sensitivity, sufficient documentation for both diagnostic and prognostic indications, and it is relatively easily performed. Negative characteristics include radiation exposure, cost, and limitations in specificity.

Stress echocardiography despite its longstanding inclusion in the relevant recommendations and guidelines is still less used. It provides increased specificity at a cost of less sensitivity, offering real-time overall heart evaluation. However, it requires dedicated expertise and is technically more demanding.

A. Methodological/Pathophysiological Considerations

Use of thallium-201 (Tl^{201}) is related with the production of low-energy photons with induction of false defects and suboptimal imaging of deep structures. Moreover, these photons are prone to scatter (induction of poor spatial resolution).

Isonitriles, which do not have redistribution, produce higher-energy photons and they can be generated onsite.

Myocardial uptake of tracers is dependent on regional perfusion and functional integrity of cardiomyocytes (1). Regional uptake may be expressed as proportion of the maximum radioactivity, thus providing a measure of perfusion on a relative scale.

Thallium-201 redistribution provides another means for relative quantitation that may be used for the interrogation of viability (2).

For semiquantitative analysis, short-axis slices of the left ventricle in four quadrants (anterior, septal, inferior, and lateral) are considered. The left ventricle is further divided into apical, mid, and basal segments. The uptake is scored in five grades: normal, mildly, moderately and severely abnormal, or absent. Standardization between individuals and centers is necessary to homogenize the analysis and integrate myocardial perfusion data, echocardiographic analysis, and cardiac magnetic resonance imaging, as it has been recently proposed in a consensus statement (3).

Commercial quantitative programs are available on most gamma camera systems (4).

They provide a quantitative estimate of the total ischemic burden and left ventricular function, employing complex algorithms, rather than relying on simple count-based programs.

For perfusion studies a "normal" database is used, and perfusion values outside the confidence limits are highlighted and thus the severity of the defect is computed. A representative practical method of evaluating the total ischemic burden is to calculate the "summed stress score" or SSS (5).

Coronary arteries presenting with a >50% diameter stenoses usually do not produce abnormal perfusion at rest (6). However, they cannot increase coronary flow postvasodilatation (either by exercise, dobutamine or dipyridamole/adenosine).

Myocardial perfusion imaging is based on the comparison of relative tracer uptake at rest and following hyperemia. Consequently, inhomogeneous coronary vasodilatation in different territories identifies indirectly coronary stenoses.

Identification of stenosis is feasible by perfusion scintigraphy when coronary flow after vasodilatation is decreased to less than half of the expected one. This may happen only in the presence of a >50% stenosis, which obviates the vasodilatory response to be more than twice the baseline flow. It should be noted that in the subtended areas by nonstenosed arteries, it usually increases fourfold.

It should be emphasized that a positive perfusion scan by any radioisotope means relative differences in the distribution of the tracer and does not require metabolic or functional ischemia (7). This is in obvious contrast to the positive outcome of the stress echo, which is always related with ischemia, being evident by myocardial systolic dysfunction.

Hyperemia may be induced either directly by coronary vasodilators or indirectly when endogenous vasodilators are produced in response to stress by exercise or dobutamine.

It should be realized that elimination of the difference in perfusion between rest and stress despite the presence of significant stenosis may be a result of specific situations such as:

1. In the case of a preexisting coronary vasodilatation due to the existing treatment and the consequent limitation of the vasodilator response.
2. In the case of a submaximal exercise.

In the aforementioned cases, the detection of less-severe stenoses is limited with a consequent lowering of the sensitivity of the perfusion test (8).

A positive result with stress echo is based upon greater increments of perfusion deficits (due to the delayed appearance of systolic dysfunction in the evolution of the ischemic cascade), then it should be expected that antianginal drug therapy might have a greater effect on the results of stress echocardiography than on perfusion imaging (9).

It should be stressed that in any functional test, the perfusion-function mismatch is less probable to occur with exercise stress because the vasodilator effect of stress is strictly related with the imposed myocardial metabolic load (heart rate–systolic blood pressure product).

B.   Diagnostic Performance of Stress Echocardiography

To simply establish the diagnosis of CAD, a qualitative assessment generally suffices. Calculation of a wall motion score adds a semiquantitative element to this assessment, which may be valuable either for prognosis, serial studies, or risk stratification with respect to the amount of myocardium in jeopardy.

The accuracy of exercise echocardiography has been examined in numerous studies (10–22). Sensitivity has ranged from a low of 71% (19) to a high of 97% (11).

There has been the expected inverse relationship between sensitivity and specificity, with specificity ranging from 64% (11), in the studies reporting the highest sensitivity, to over 90% (19) in studies with lower sensitivity.

The sensitivity for detection of patients with single-vessel disease has been lower (59–94%) than sensitivity for detection of patients with multivessel disease (85–100%).

Although the sensitivity for identifying patients with multivessel disease is high, it is common to underestimate the number of diseased vessels. This is due when a diagnostic test is stopped for an indication such as angina or ST-segment depression. Thus, the most critical lesion becomes unmasked and less severe stenoses may not be detected.

A similar level of accuracy with many of the same limitations has been noted for dobutamine stress echocardiography (23–28).

The definition of "significant" stenosis affects diagnostic accuracy. Sensitivity is greatest when significant stenosis is defined as a threshold of >70% compared to >50% diameter stenosis.

The accuracy of stress echocardiography will be adversely affected in the presence of microvascular disease, in the case of an acute hypertensive response to stress, and when a significant left ventricular hypertrophy is present, especially with concentric remodeling (combination of increased wall thickness with normal or small chamber sizes). In this situation, wall stress is reduced, and the likelihood of a false-negative result is increased.

The ability to precisely identify significant stenosis in the left anterior descending artery has exceeded that for the posterior circulation. This is due to the greater ease of the left anterior descending territory interrogation compared with the evaluation of the posterior endocardium, as well as with the greater territories supplied by the anterior circulation. Because of the overlap between the right coronary artery and circumflex coronary artery territories, precise separation of these territories is not feasible.

Accuracy is affected by delayed imaging, by the suboptimal image quality, and by a low level of physical stress, resulting in a suboptimal cardiovascular workload, resulting in a reduction in sensitivity. The degree to which a suboptimal heart rate impacts the accuracy of pharmacological stress is less clear. Vasodilator stress does not rely on increased workload and traditional estimates of workload may have little relevance. Dobutamine increases the heart rate and blood pressure and has a great effect on contractility, which drives myocardial oxygen demand, all of which mimic the effects of exercise. Thus, a "suboptimal" heart rate response to dobutamine, if seen in the presence of a hypercontractile response, may not confer as great a decrement in accuracy as a proportional reduction in heart rate during physical stress.

C. The Issue of the Type of Stress

Physical Exercise

A meta-analysis suggested similar sensitivity for stress echocardiography and myocardial scintigraphy, with a higher specificity found with stress echocardiography (29). In pooled data weighted by the sample size of each study (29), exercise echocardiography had a sensitivity of 85% [95% confidence interval (CI), 83–87%] with a specificity of 77% (95% CI, 74–80%). Exercise single-photon emission computed tomography (SPECT) yielded a similar sensitivity of 87% (95% CI, 86–88%) but a lower specificity of 64% (95% CI, 60–68%).

In a model comparing exercise echocardiography to exercise SPECT, exercise echocardiography was associated with significantly better discriminatory power (parameter estimate, 1.18; 95% CI, 0.71–1.65), when adjusted for age, publication year, and a setting including known CAD for SPECT studies.

In models comparing the discriminatory abilities of exercise, echocardiography and exercise SPECT versus exercise testing without imaging, both exercise echocardiography and SPECT performed significantly better than exercise testing. The incremental improvement in performance was greater for exercise echocardiography (3.43; 95% CI, 2.74–4.11) than for SPECT (1.49; 95% CI, 0.91–2.08) (29).

The validation studies of stress echocardiography are subjected to the same issues of referral (probability for existing significant disease) and test verification bias (further performance of coronary angiography) as other techniques. The combination of referral and verification bias typically leads to an overstatement of sensitivity in early studies. After adjustment for referral and verification bias, sensitivities typically are lower and specificity higher in the unselected general population than reported in the initial verification cohorts (21).

Pharmacological Stress

In meta-analysis including 82 studies (30), it was found that vasodilator SPECT imaging had higher sensitivity but lower specificity than did vasodilator echocardiography. Dobutamine SPECT imaging had similar sensitivity but lower specificity than did dobutamine echocardiography. In the same study, of the three pharmacological stressors, dipyridamole was the most commonly combined with SPECT imaging. SPECT studies used either thallium or sestamibi as the nuclear isotope. The two isotopes had similar sensitivities and specificities for all pharmacological stressors. The sensitivity and specificity of dipyridamole SPECT imaging were not significantly different from those of adenosine SPECT imaging. In contrast, most of the studies of dobutamine SPECT studies used sestamibi as the imaging agent. Compared with studies of vasodilator SPECT, dobutamine SPECT studies had a lower sensitivity but similar specificity. In contrast, of the three pharmacologic stressors, dobutamine was the most commonly combined with echocardiography. Dobutamine echocardiography had a higher sensitivity but a lower specificity than did dipyridamole or adenosine echocardiography.

When echocardiographic and SPECT vasodilator studies are compared, adenosine and dipyridamole SPECT studies offered the highest sensitivities 90% and 89%, respectively. Adenosine and dipyridamole echocardiographic studies offered the highest specificities, 91% and 93%, respectively. Choice of the imaging modality for vasodilator studies seems to involve a trade off of higher sensitivity or specificity.

The results with dobutamine are significantly different than the results with the vasodilators.

Dobutamine echocardiography and SPECT results are comparable with the results from a previous study of exercise echocardiography and SPECT imaging (29).

The sensitivities of dobutamine echocardiography (80%) and dobutamine SPECT imaging (82%) are similar, as are the sensitivities of exercise echocardiography (85%) and exercise SPECT imaging (87%). Similarly, the specificity of dobutamine echocardiography (84%) is higher than that of dobutamine SPECT imaging (75%), and the specificity of exercise echocardiography (77%) is higher than that of exercise SPECT imaging (64%). This suggests that echocardiography may be a better myocardial imaging modality for both dobutamine and exercise studies.

Exercise studies offer a slightly higher sensitivity and a lower specificity than dobutamine studies. Of course, only exercise studies offer functional data.

The results in the sex subanalysis are limited by the fact that few studies presented sex-specific data. However, dobutamine echocardiography had a similar sensitivity and specificity in women and men, a finding that had also been confirmed in exercise echocardiographic studies (31).

D. The Issue of the Extent of Coronary Artery Disease

The finding of imaging abnormalities in >2 vascular territories appears to be a specific, although not sensitive criterion for the detection of multivessel disease. In clinical practice, the degree of abnormality on the imaging study is often as important as whether a study is "positive" or "negative."

In a meta-analysis (30), the issue of multivessel disease was analyzed in two ways. First, it was considered only whether the noninvasive test showed any imaging abnormality in the presence of multivessel disease. In this instance, the number of vascular territories identified was not taken into account. Thus, a study showing only a lateral wall motion abnormality in a subject with triple-vessel disease would count as a true-positive test. The vast majority of the studies used this definition. The second definition of multivessel disease required that noninvasive imaging showed abnormalities in ≥2 vascular territories in order to be considered positive for the presence of multivessel disease. Thus, a study with a lateral wall motion abnormality in a patient with triple-vessel disease would be considered as being negative. At least two coronary territories would have to be abnormal in this case for the study to be positive. However, in this scenario, exact matching of the abnormal imaging areas to the diseased vessels is not required.

This allows the evaluation of the sensitivity and specificity per coronary territories and not only per patients as in the first definition. Fewer studies presented data in this format. As expected, the sensitivity calculated by the use of this definition for the detection of multivessel disease is significantly lower than the less exact first definition. However, the specificity of finding abnormalities in >2 coronary territories compares favorably with the specificities for the detection of CAD in general (per patient).

E. Selecting the Stressor in Clinical Practice

In particular, dipyridamole and dobutamine nuclear imaging studies have higher specificities for multivessel CAD detection than they do for general CAD detection. Thus, the presence of multiple imaging abnormalities seems to be a specific but not a sensitive marker of multivessel disease. It seems that extensive imaging abnormality, if present, is a reliable sign of more extensive underlying disease, especially in nuclear imaging studies.

Maximum specificity can be attained by the use of a vasodilator with echocardiography. Maximum sensitivity can be attained by the use of a vasodilator combined with nuclear imaging. Dobutamine echocardiography offers a good compromise between sensitivity and specificity. The clinician can customize the test selection to the clinical situation.

F. Specific Practical Considerations

Breast and diaphragmatic attenuation are usual causes of difficulties in nuclear imaging. Due to attenuation, the posterior wall remains difficult to be assessed by perfusion scintigraphy. In contrast, echocardiography may underestimate dyssynergies of the lateral wall due to the "side lobe" effects and the overlying lung, and thus scintigraphy may be more accurate in the lateral segments (32).

Stress echocardiography and myocardial scintigraphy seek different end points (ventricular dyssynergy and perfusion abnormalities, respectively), but with a common target—the identification of significant epicardial coronary artery stenosis.

Patients with perfusion abnormalities (positive scintigraphy) and no ventricular dyssynergy (negative echocardiography) might have an imbalance efficient enough to induce perfusion abnormalities but not to reveal wall dyssynergy. Whether there is heterogeneity of perfusion with not even a trace of ischemia (wall dyssynergy) or with dyssynergy that is too small or too brief to be detected by current echocardiographic methodology cannot be proven. It has been suggested that the presence or the absence of left ventricular wall dyssynergy during dobutamine infusion is not related to the extension of perfusion abnormalities (33).

The equivalence in the diagnostic accuracy of stress echocardiography and myocardial perfusion imaging might be surprising considering the ischemic cascade in which perfusion disturbances precede ischemia, thus supporting perfusion imaging to be more sensitive modality than wall motion dyssynergies for the detection of ischemia. Outcome of the noninvasive tests are affected not only by the underlying pathophysiology, but also by the physical characteristics of the imaging modalities themselves. The physical strengths of echocardiography (spatial and temporal resolution) combined with the experienced assessment of segmental wall thickening may overcome for the delayed appearance of systolic dysfunction on the time domain of the ischemic cascade.

G. Specific Clinical Entities to be Studied by Stress Echocardiography

The accuracy of the imaging techniques and especially the specificity is affected in women (34), patients with left bundle branch block (LBBB) (35), and left ventricular hypertrophy (36) (Table 1).

Breast attenuation artefacts occur often in the unprocessed SPECT data, and adoption of a higher threshold may reduce the sensitivity, especially in small female hearts (34).

When stress echocardiography is used in LBBB, the test is accurate in the territories of the circumflex and right coronary arteries. However, sensitivity may be decreased in the presence of left ventricular enlargement (37). Perfusion imaging has false-positive perfusion defects in the septum due to altered regional blood supply as a result of delayed septal activation that are heart rate dependent. Despite the use of adenosine, which does not increase heart rate significantly, the issue remains unresolved (38).

Left ventricular hypertrophy is related with heterogeneity of regional flow reserve due to inadequate growth of the coronary vasculature, alterations of

TABLE 1 Stress Echocardiography Vs. Radionuclide Imaging: Test Selection[a]

Stress echocardiography is more useful in:
1. Left ventricular hypertrophy and left bundle branch block.
2. Patients with expected severe ischemia or unstable, since ischemia may be detected earlier due to the continuous echocardiographic monitoring of regional myocardial function.
3. Patients with known coronary artery disease to evaluate the adequacy of treatment, as stress echocardiography detects directly ischemic insult on myocardial performance than perfusion heterogeneity.
4. Patients with coexistent valve dysfunction or other cardiac structural pathology.

Perfusion is more useful in:
1. Postinfarction patients: easy assess of combined ischemia-scar, avoidance of tethering effect by echocardiography.
2. Patients unable to exercise and with contraindications to dobutamine, since vasodilatory echocardiography is less sensitive in one-vessel disease.
3. Poor echocardiographic windows.

---

[a]The combination of stress echocardiography and perfusion imaging cannot be recommended because of cost constraints.

vascular geometry, and rearrangement of microvascular resistance, resulting in augmentation of resting myocardial blood flow (39). The accuracy of stress echocardiography in these conditions is not seriously compromised (31,40), with the unique exception of hypertrophied ventricles with concentric remodeling (41).

The agreement between echocardiography and perfusion scintigraphy is decreased to a 70% to 80% for the specific identification of normal, ischemic, or infarcted myocardium (42). Resting akinesis at echocardiography may be due to tethering of normal myocardium due to adjacent zone with scar, stunning, or hibernation and not only infarction. Thus, discordant outcome between stress echocardiography and myocardial scintigraphy might be increased in the infarct zones.

The detection of ischemia within areas of resting wall motion abnormalities is usually easier with nuclear imaging.

It should be stressed that the final clarification of equivocal cases for scar should not rely on coronary angiography, which does not contribute to the evaluation of the myocardial integrity.

II. RISK STRATIFICATION IN CORONARY ARTERY DISEASE

A. Role of SPECT

Normal Perfusion Scan

A normal stress thallium-201 study has independent prognostic value (43).

A 6-year follow up study of normal thallium-201 perfusion studies (on 1137 patients) showed that the cardiac event rate (nonfatal myocardial infarction or cardiac death) was only 0.88% (44).

In the presence of a normal stress myocardial perfusion scan, exercise ECG had no added prognostic value (45,46).

Technetium-99 m sestamibi has been found to have a similar prognostic value.

A review of 14 trials including over 12,000 patients with stable chest pain confirmed that normal technetium 99 m-sestamibi SPECT is associated with a hard cardiac event rate of 0.6% per year (47).

Abnormal Perfusion Scan

As the myocardial perfusion scan represents global left ventricular perfusion, the size, severity, and reversibility of the defect implies the extent of risk, or the "total ischemic burden." The number of segments involved on a multislice tomographic evaluation of the SPECT study can be used to calculate both the extent and severity of the ischemic myocardium.

In large studies (over 20,000 patients), the SSS score predicted patient outcome. A normal SSS (0–3) was associated with a mortality of less than 1%, whereas an increasing SSS predicted higher cardiac mortality (45).

Myocardial perfusion scintigraphy provided additional incremental prognostic value irrespective of the Duke treadmill score result (45).

In lower risk scans (mildly abnormal; SSS 4–8), there was no survival advantage for revascularization. However, as the size of the defect increased (SSS > 9), the advantage with revascularization showed an increased survival benefit (48).

This has important implications for the treatment provided and the costs associated with it. However, it should be stressed that apart from the extent of ischemia expressed as SSS score, prognosis using myocardial scintigraphy is decisively ominous only when additional information for left ventricular dysfunction is evident.

Indirect information of left ventricular systolic dysfunction by myocardial scintigraphy is provided by the presence of left ventricular chamber dilatation postexercise and increased lung uptake with thallium-201.

It should be noted that stress echocardiography provides a direct evaluation of regional myocardial dysfunction due to underlying respective ischemia, thus being theoretically more coherent to overall left ventricular dysfunction and prognosis.

B. Role of Stress Echocardiography

In patients with known or suspected CAD, regional and global ventricular function at peak exercise is a predictor of subsequent cardiac events and is additive to clinical variables, exercise duration, ECG changes, and resting ventricular function (49–51). This prognostic yield is also important in hypertension and diabetes mellitus, and it remains independent of age or gender.

An exercise wall motion score index >1.4 or exercise ejection fraction <50% have a similar prognostic yield to that of a myocardial perfusion defect size of <15% (49).

Exercise echocardiography can further stratify cardiac risk events when combined to the Duke treadmill score (50).

A risk index combining echocardiographic and exercise variables improves the risk stratification of exercise echocardiography, particularly its negative predictive value for cardiac events (52).

Incidence of cardiac events in the presence of a normal exercise echocardiogram and good exercise tolerance is usually <1% per year (49–52).

Similar to exercise echocardiography, pharmacological stress with either dobutamine or dipyridamole has been shown to have significant prognostic power (53–56). As it can be anticipated, a greater extent of segmental dysfunction, acute dilation of the left ventricle at maximal stress implying an increased enddiastolic pressure, and a low ischemic threshold are related with a worse outcome.

A normal dobutamine stress echocardiogram reassures a low spontaneous cardiovascular event rate (usually <1.5% per year) (53–56).

C. Specific Cohorts: Prognosis After Acute Myocardial Infarction

Similar principles apply to the evaluation of risk after myocardial infarction.

In meta-analysis myocardial scintigraphy and stress echocardiography have comparable prognostic value (57). Identification of high-risk patients after an acute myocardial infarction should include clinical features such as recurrent postinfarction angina, older age, and heart failure.

After infarction, worsening ventricular function during stress is related with a worse prognosis. The extent of resting dyssynergies, the extent of inducible ischemia, and the absence of viability are related with a worse prognosis (58–60).

D. Cardiac Risk Stratification in Major Surgery

For preoperative risk stratification, the application of a functional test is advised when an intermediate risk for significant CAD is present.

When a myocardial perfusion test is positive, the perioperative risk is at least moderate, especially when the extent of ischemia is great, or an additional stress echocardiographic evaluation reveals extensive systolic dysfunction with a low threshold. In such circumstances revascularization before surgery might be considered (61).

By definition, a vascular surgery itself represents a major risk factor for CAD with a high probability for coexistence of significant CAD.

In meta-analysis, both myocardial scintigraphy and stress echocardiography have equal prognostic contribution for perioperative risk assessment (62,63) (see also Chap. 11).

III. DETECTION OF MYOCARDIAL VIABILITY

A. Role of Stress Echocardiography and Myocardial Scintigraphy

The criteria to define "viability" are not based on an independent gold standard of myocardial viable tissue, but they are empirically accepted on the basis of the detection of the myocardial segments that expresses functional (systolic) recovery following effective revascularization.

Both stress echocardiography and myocardial perfusion scintigraphy may be used for the detection of viable myocardium. The detection of viable tissue is dependent on the presence of contractile reserve and the identification of cell membrane integrity. Viability response by both tests is inversely proportional to the presence and transmural extent of myocardial fibrosis (64).

It should be realized that regional thickening reflects the function of the subendocardial zone itself, with a very limited or absent contribution of the outermost subepicardial zone (65).

B. Accuracy for the Detection of Viable Myocardium

The accuracy of stress echocardiography and myocardial perfusion scintigraphy for the prediction of myocardial functional recovery has been proven.

A higher sensitivity for scintigraphy with a greater specificity of echocardiography has been detected (66–69).

However, it should be clarified that many of these so-called false-positive segments with scintigraphy might reflect situations where viable tissue is truly present but it does not contribute to the regional thickening either due to a limited amount or due to a subepicardial localization.

Chronic systolic ventricular dysfunction does not necessarily imply irreversible myocardial injury. Indicators of myocardial viability and potential systolic recovery have included contractile reserve to inotropic stimulation and preserved myocardial thickness, as well as intact myocardial perfusion and metabolism. Incremental infusion of dobutamine elicits an augmentation of regional function in dysfunctional segments that is predictive of recovery of function after revascularization (70,71).

The use of high-dose in addition to low-dose dobutamine may categorize the responses for contractile reserve, with significant implications for both recovery of function after revascularization and prognosis.

Dysfunctional myocardium shows one of four responses to dobutamine:

(1)   biphasic response: augmentation at a low dose followed by deterioration at a higher dose;
(2)   sustained improvement: improvement in function at a low dose that persists or further improves at higher doses;
(3)   worsening of function, without contractile reserve; and
(4)   no change in function.

Sensitivity for recovery of function ranges between 74% and 88%, with a specificity between 73% and 87% (71). A biphasic response has the best predictive value for recovery of function after revascularization.

A combination of the types of responses to dobutamine (e.g., any contractile reserve) increases the sensitivity of dobutamine stress echocardiography with a slight decrease in specificity for predicting recovery of function.

Comparison of the determination of viability with dobutamine stress echocardiography and radionuclide studies has shown higher sensitivity and lower specificity for radionuclide techniques (68,71).

Myocardial thickness represents a specific indicator of myocardial viability. Myocardium that is thin (<6 mm) has a very low likelihood of recovery of function after revascularization (negative predictive value of 93%). Combined contractile reserve during dobutamine stress echocardiography and preserved myocardial thickness (>6 mm) yields the best diagnostic accuracy for echocardiography in predicting recovery of function (72,73).

Observational data suggest that dysfunctional but viable myocardium that is not revascularized constitutes a predictor of further ischemic events and higher overall mortality. Recent studies using dobutamine stress echocardiography have demonstrated a very poor prognosis in individuals with depressed ventricular function who have no evidence of myocardial viability, irrespective of whether or not they underwent revascularization. Best prognosis was observed in patients with evidence of myocardial viability who underwent revascularization (71,74).

C. Prediction of Functional Recovery

Improvements in ejection fraction, functional capacity, quality of life, and survival are not proportional to the amount of viable tissue detected by any method.

A critical amount of viable tissue (at least 4 out of 16 left ventricular segments) is required to be detected in order to guarantee an improvement of global left ventricular function (ejection fraction increase >5%) (75).

A similar extent of viability is required when nuclear perfusion imaging has been used (76).

Moreover, there are proposals that resting improvement might not be apparent despite the evidence of inotropic reserve revealed by the low-dose dobutamine provocation following a successful revascularization (77).

D. Prognostic Implications

Observational studies of medically treated patients with viable myocardium detected with either stress echocardiography or myocardial scintigraphy have shown that the event rate over 1 to 2 years of follow-up is increased compared to revascularized patients. In meta-analysis (78), the tests have been proven to be equipotent for risk stratification.

The amount of viable tissue detected by either test is related to the improvement in ejection fraction, and the reduction of risk with revascularization is related to the extent of viability (79).

IV. PREDICTION OF CARDIAC EVENTS IN CHRONIC STABLE CORONARY ARTERY DISEASE

The yearly event rate (death or hard events) with a negative stress imaging test is less than 1% per year for at least the first 2 years and probably 4 to 5 years— events later in follow-up probably reflect the presence of progressive coronary disease (51,80–82).

Patients liable to events despite a normal scan include those at high pretest risk (e.g., the elderly, diabetic subjects unable to exercise) (83) and situations where a false-negative interpretation is possible (e.g., those undergoing insufficient stress, angina despite the absence of imaging abnormalities) (51).

For both echocardiography and nuclear tests, the next step in a patient with a positive test is to substratify the level of risk. Clinical features such as age, diabetes, and symptoms of congestive heart failure are predictive of outcome in stable CAD (84) and may be used to select patients for more extensive testing and combined imaging assessment.

Both stress echocardiography (50) and myocardial perfusion SPECT (85) appear to be equally useful in substratifying patients at intermediate risk of events.

The total extent and severity of abnormal perfusion (SSS) or abnormal function (53) are predictive of outcome.

The evidence based on nuclear imaging is greater in this respect—a number of studies have confirmed that the frequency of adverse outcomes in patients with mild fixed or reversible defects is low and does not justify intervention.

Ischemic threshold is analogous to the heart rate at the onset of ST-segment depression and may be assessed with pharmacological and bicycle stress echocardiography. Patients developing ischemia at a low heart rate are more likely to have events than those in whom ischemia is induced only at peak stress (61).

A. Implications of Risk Stratification Data for Patient Management

The contemporary use of functional testing has been focused not exclusively to the diagnosis of CAD but in addition to the refinement of risk stratification and consequent decision making for treatment strategies.

It is of great importance to interrogate and justify not only the presence of ischemia but also the territories involved in the exact location and the respective extent of ischemia. In these respects, consideration only of the sensitivity and specificity for the diagnosis of coronary disease is of limited relevance.

The regional accuracy of stress echocardiography and perfusion scintigraphy can generally be expected to be similar.

The assessment of the extent of ischemia is equipotent with both imaging modalities.

In the recent guidelines for percutaneous coronary interventions and specifically for management of acute coronary syndromes, both stress echocardiography and myocardial scintigraphy may be used interchangeably for risk stratification (86). Thus, it is imperative to support the use of the functional tests in the stable chronic artery disease patients.

The reliability of both echocardiographic and nuclear imaging is dependent upon expertise. Since both modalities share similar accuracy and ability for risk stratification and decision-making management, then the local expertise should be taken into account.

Echocardiography is clinically more relevant especially when nonischemic aspects are of interest (e.g., anatomical assessment for valvular/pericardial disease, ventricular hypertrophy, heart failure), and it is better with respect to cost and versatility.

Nuclear imaging might be more useful in unstable patients (because vasodilatory stressors provoke less ischemia) and in patients with prior infarction.

V. FINANCIAL ASPECT: BALANCING COST AND TEST ACCURACY

The simplest approach to cost control with functional testing is to examine the relationship between the number of diagnoses missed and the total cost of testing (including that of coronary angiography, assuming it will be applied in all positive outcomes). Thus, the performance of stress echocardiography as an initial test in some subgroups—for example, women and patients with LV hypertrophy (18,19)—is justified on the basis of fewer false-positive results and therefore unnecessary angiograms.

A more complicated approach is to anticipate that the treatment of properly diagnosed disease improves both the quality of life and the survival. One modeling approach (87) anticipated that the diagnosis of significant coronary disease improves life expectancy at full life quality by 3 years over a 10-year follow-up. With this analysis, the most inexpensive test was exercise echocardiography due to its high specificity.

However, accounting only for the anticipated improvements in outcome, the most effective test seems to be direct coronary angiography due to its optimal sensitivity. Thus, patients at low-to-intermediate probability (20–50%) of significant coronary disease are optimally studied by exercise echocardiography. In this scenario, the numbers of positive tests could be expected to be low (resulting in small improvement in life expectancy when corrected properly), and the high specificity of the test controlled the number of angiograms (and thus decreasing the key component of the cost). In contrast, individuals at intermediate-to-high probability of disease (50–80%) were most efficiently studied by SPECT.

Kuntz et al. (88) concluded that reasonable cost-effectiveness could be attained with exercise ECG or exercise echocardiography in patients at mild-to-moderate risk for CAD, and coronary angiography in patients with a high pretest probability of disease. Nonetheless, the major methodological issue with this kind of analysis is that the prognostic value of diagnosing disease is highly variable and often quite limited. Thus, models based upon observed outcomes should be applied.

The END (economics of noninvasive diagnosis) study (89) compared direct cardiac catheterization with SPECT followed by selective cardiac catheterization to diagnose CAD in specialist cardiology centers in the United States.

None of the patients underwent risk stratification with the standard exercise ECG. Diagnostic and follow up costs were lower when a strategy employing SPECT before selective cardiac catheterization was used. The cardiac deaths and nonfatal myocardial infarction rates were slightly lower in the SPECT arm than in the direct catheterization arm, at 2.8% and 2.8% versus 3.3% and 3.0%, respectively ($p =$ ns).

The EMPIRE (economics of myocardial perfusion imaging in Europe) study (90) compared 396 patient records from eight hospitals in four European countries. Retrospective analysis on suitable patients was done to compare four different strategies used to diagnose CAD. The results suggested that a strategy using SPECT was economically efficient without any effect on the outcome for the patient.

In a recent study (91), they examined prognosis and cost-effectiveness of exercise echocardiography versus SPECT imaging in stable, intermediate risk, chest pain patients. Cox proportional hazard models were employed to assess time to cardiac death or myocardial infarction. Total cardiovascular costs were summed (discounted and inflation-corrected) throughout follow-up. A cost-effectiveness ratio <$50,000 per life year saved (LYS) was considered favorable for economic efficiency. The risk-adjusted 3-year death or myocardial infarction rates classified by extent of ischemia were similar, ranging from 2.3% to 8.0% for echocardiography and from 3.5% to 11.0% for SPECT. Cost-effectiveness ratios for echocardiography were <$20,000/LYS when the annual risk of death or myocardial infarction was >2%. However, when yearly cardiac event rate were >2%, cost-effectiveness ratios for echocardiography versus SPECT were in the range of $66,686/LYS to $419,522/LYS. For patients with established coronary disease (i.e., ≥2% annual event risk), SPECT ischemia was associated with earlier and greater utilization of coronary revascularization resulting in an incremental cost-effectiveness ratio of $32,381/LYS. This study suggested that a strategy aimed at cost-effective testing would support using echocardiography in low-risk patients with suspected coronary disease, whereas higher risk patients benefit from referral to SPECT imaging.

REFERENCES

1. Maddahi J, Rodrigues E, Berman DS, et al. State of the art myocardial perfusion imaging. In: Verani MS, ed. Nuclear Cardiology: State of the Art. Philadelphia, PA: W. B. Saunders, 1994:199–222.
2. Dilsizian V, Rocco TP, Freedman NM, et al. Enhanced detection of ischemic hut viable myocardium by the reinjection of thallium after stress-redistribution imaging. N Engl J Med 1990; 323:141–146.
3. Cerqueira MD, Weissman NJ, Dilsizian V, et al. Standardized myocardial segmentation and nomenclature for tomographic imaging of the heart: A statement for healthcare professionals from the cardiac imaging committee of the Council on Clinical Cardiology of the American Heart Association. J Nucl Cardiol 2002; 9:240–245.
4. Faber TL, Cooke CD, Folks RD, et al. Left ventricular function and perfusion from gated SPECT perfusion images: An integrated method. J Nucl Med 1999; 40:650–659.
5. Berman D, Hachamovitch R, Lewin H, et al. Risk stratification in coronary artery disease: Implications for stabilization and prevention. Am J Cardiol 1997; 79:10–16.
6. Gould KL, Westcott RJ, Albro PC, et al. Noninvasive assessment of coronary stenoses by myocardial imaging during pharmacologic coronary vasodilatation. II. Clinical methodology and feasibility. Am J Cardiol 1978; 41:279–287.
7. Fragasso G, Lu C, Dabrowski P, et al. Comparison of stress/rest myocardial perfusion tomography, dipyridamole and dobutamine stress echocardiography for the detection of coronary disease in hypertensive patients with chest pain and positive exercise test. J Am Coll Cardiol 1999; 34:441–447.
8. Iskandrian AS, Heo J, Kong B, et al. Effect of exercise level on the ability of thallium-201 tomographic imaging in detecting coronary artery disease: Analysis of 461 patients. J Am Coll Cardiol 1989; 14:1477–1486.
9. Lattanzi F, Picano E, Bolognese L, et al. Inhibition of dipyridamole-induced ischemia by antianginal therapy in humans. Correlation with exercise electrocardiography. Circulation 1991; 83:1256–1262.
10. Armstrong WF, O'Donnell J, Ryan T, et al. Effect of prior myocardial infarction and extent and location of coronary disease on accuracy of exercise echocardiography. J Am Coll Cardiol 1987; 10:531–538.
11. Crouse LJ, Harbrecht JJ, Vacek JL, et al. Exercise echocardiography as a screening test for coronary artery disease and correlation with coronary arteriography. Am J Cardiol 1991; 67:1213–1218.
12. Marwick TH, Nemec JJ, Pashkow FJ, et al. Accuracy and limitations of exercise echocardiography in a routine clinical setting. J Am Coll Cardiol 1992; 19:74–81.
13. Quinones MA, Verani MS, Haichin RM, et al. Exercise echocardiography versus 201Tl single-photon emission computed tomography in evaluation of coronary artery disease: Analysis of 292 patients. Circulation 1992; 85:1026–1031.
14. Hecht HS, DeBord L, Shaw R, et al. Digital supine bicycle stress echocardiography: A new technique for evaluating coronary artery disease. J Am Coll Cardiol 1993; 21:950–956.
15. Roger VL, Pellikka PA, Oh JK, et al. Identification of multivessel coronary artery disease by exercise echocardiography. J Am Coll Cardiol 1994; 24:109–114.
16. Beleslin BD, Ostojic M, Stepanovic J, et al. Stress echocardiography in the detection of myocardial ischemia: Head-to-head comparison of exercise, dobutamine, and dipyridamole tests. Circulation 1994; 90:1168–1176.
17. Roger VL, Pellikka PA, Oh JK, et al. Stress echocardiography. Part I. Exercise echocardiography: Techniques, implementation, clinical applications, and correlations. Mayo Clin Proc 1995; 70:5–15.
18. Marwick TH, Anderson T, Williams MJ, et al. Exercise echocardiography is an accurate and cost-efficient technique for detection of coronary artery disease in women. J Am Coll Cardiol 1995; 26:335–341.

19. Marwick TH, Torelli J, Harjai K, et al. Influence of left ventricular hypertrophy on detection of coronary artery disease using exercise echocardiography. J Am Coll Cardiol 1995; 26:1180–1186.
20. Luotolahti TH, Torelli J, Hartiala J. Exercise echocardiography in the diagnosis of coronary artery disease. Ann Med 1996; 28:73–77.
21. Roger VL, Pellikka PA, Bell MR, et al. Sex and test verification bias: Impact on the diagnostic value of exercise echocardiography. Circulation 1997; 95:405–410.
22. Badruddin SM, Ahmad A, Mickelson J, et al. Supine bicycle versus post-treadmill exercise echocardiography in the detection of myocardial ischemia: A randomized single-blind cross-over trial. J Am Coll Cardiol 1999; 33:1485–1490.
23. Segar DS, Brown SE, Sawada SG, et al. Dobutamine stress echocardiography: Correlation with coronary lesion severity as determined by quantitative angiography. J Am Coll Cardiol 1992; 19:1197–1202.
24. Marcovitz PA, Armstrong WF. Accuracy of dobutamine stress echocardiography in detecting coronary artery disease. Am J Cardiol 1992; 69:1269–1273.
25. McNeill AJ, Fioretti PM, el-Said SM, et al. Enhanced sensitivity for detection of coronary artery disease by addition of atropine to dobutamine stress echocardiography. Am J Cardiol 1992; 70:41–46.
26. Marwick T, D'Hondt AM, Baudhuin T, et al. Optimal use of dobutamine stress for the detection and evaluation of coronary artery disease: Combination with echocardiography or scintigraphy, or both? J Am Coll Cardiol 1993; 22:159–167.
27. Previtali M, Lanzarini L, Fetiveau R, et al. Comparison of dobutamine stress echocardiography, dipyridamole stress echocardiography and exercise stress testing for diagnosis of coronary artery disease. Am J Cardiol 1993; 72:865–870.
28. Takeuchi M, Araki M, Nakashima Y, et al. Comparison of dobutamine stress echocardiography and stress thallium-201 single photon emission computed tomography for detecting coronary artery disease. J Am Soc Echocardiogr 1993; 6:593–602.
29. Fleischmann KE, Hunink MG, Kuntz KM, et al. Exercise echocardiography or exercise SPECT imaging? A meta-analysis of diagnostic test performance. JAMA 1998; 280:913–920.
30. Kwok Y, Kim C, Grady D, et al. Meta-analysis of exercise testing to detect coronary artery disease in women. Am J Cardiol 1999; 83:660–666.
31. Kim C, Kwok Y, Heagerty P, et al. Pharmacologic stress testing for coronary disease diagnosis: A meta-analysis. Am Heart J 2001; 142:934–944.
32. Pozzoli MM, Fioretti PM, Salustri A, et al. Exercise echocardiography and technetium 99 m MIBI single photon emission computed tomography in the detection of coronary artery disease. Am J Cardiol 1991; 67:350–355.
33. Elhendy A, Geleijnse ML, Roelandt JR, et al. Dobutamine induced hypoperfusion without transient wall motion abnormalities: Less severe ischemia or less severe stress? J Am Coll Cardiol 1996; 27:323–329.
34. Hansen CL, Crabbe D, Rubin D, et al. Lower diagnostic accuracy of thallium-201 SPECT myocardial perfusion imaging in women: An effect of smaller chamber size. J Am Coll Cardiol 1996; 28:1214–1219.
35. DePuey EG, Guertler-Krawczynska B, Robbins WL. Thallium-201 SPECT in coronary disease patients with left bundle branch block. J Nucl Med 1998; 29:1479–1485.
36. Houghton TL, Frank MI, Carr AA, et al. Relations among impaired coronary flow reserve, left ventricular hypertrophy, and thallium perfusion defects in hypertensive patients without obstructive coronary artery disease. J Am Coll Cardiol 1990; 15:43–51.
37. Geleijnse ML, Vigna C, Kasprzak JD, et al. Usefulness and limitations of dobutamine-atropine stress echocardiography for the diagnosis of coronary artery disease in patients with left bundle branch block. A multicentre study. Eur Heart J 2000; 21(20):1666–1673.
38. O'Keefe JH Jr, Bateman TM, Barnhart CS. Adenosine thallium-201 is superior to exercise thallium-201 for detecting coronary artery disease in patients with left bundle branch block. J Am Coll Cardiol 1993; 21(6):1332–1338.
39. O'Keefe DD, Hoffman JI, Cheitlin R, et al. Coronary blood flow in experimental canine left ventricular hypertrophy. Circ Res 1978; 43(1):43–51.

40. Mairesse GH, Marwick TH, Arnese M, et al. Improved identification of coronary artery disease in patients with left bundle branch block by use of dobutamine stress echocardiography and comparison with myocardial perfusion tomography. Am J Cardiol 1995; 76:321–325.

41. Smart SC, Knickelbine T, Malik F, et al. Dobutamine-atropine stress echocardiography for the detection of coronary artery disease in patients with left ventricular hypertrophy. Importance of chamber size and systolic wall stress. Circulation 2000; 101: 258–263.

42. Marwick TH, Nemec II, Stewart WJ, et al. Diagnosis of coronary artery disease using exercise echocardiography and positron emission tomography: Comparison and analysis of discrepant results. J Am Soc Echocardiogr 1992; 5:231–238.

43. Wahl JM, Hakki AH, Iskandrian AS. Prognostic implications of normal exercise thallium 201 images. Arch Intern Med 1985; 145:253–256.

44. Vanzetto G, Ormezzano O, Fagret D, et al. Long-term additive prognostic value of thallium-201 myocardial perfusion imaging over clinical and exercise stress test in low to intermediate risk patients: Study in 1137 patients with 6-year follow-up. Circulation 1999; 100:1521–1527.

45. Hachamovitch R, Berman DS, Kiat H, et al. Exercise myocardial perfusion SPECT in patients without known coronary artery disease: Incremental prognostic value and use in risk stratification. Circulation 1996; 93:905–914.

46. Taillefer R, DePuey EG, Udelson JE, et al. Comparative diagnostic accuracy of Tl-201 and Tc-99 m sestamibi SPECT imaging (perfusion and ECG-gated SPECT) in detecting coronary artery disease in women. J Am Coll Cardiol 1997; 29:69–77.

47. Iskander S, Iskandrian AE. Risk assessment using single-photon emission computed tomographic technetium-99 m sestamibi imaging. J Am Coll Cardiol 1998; 32:57–62.

48. Hachamovitch R, Berman DS, Shaw LJ, et al. Incremental prognostic value of myocardial perfusion single photon emission computed tomography for the prediction of cardiac death: Differential stratification for risk of cardiac death and myocardial. Circulation 1998; 97:535–543.

49. Olmos LI, Dakik H, Gordon R, et al. Long-term prognostic value of exercise echocardiography compared with exercise 201Tl, ECG, and clinical variables in patients evaluated for coronary artery disease. Circulation 1998; 98:2679–2686.

50. Marwick TH, Case C, Vasey C, et al. Prediction of mortality by exercise echocardiography: A strategy for combination with the Duke treadmill score. Circulation 2001; 103:2566–2571.

51. McCully RB, Roger VL, Mahoney DW, et al. Outcome after normal exercise echocardiography and predictors of subsequent cardiac events: Follow-up of 1325 patients. J Am Coll Cardiol 1998; 31:144–149.

52. Mazur W, Rivera JM, Khoury AF, et al. Prognostic value of exercise echocardiography: Validation of a new risk index combining echocardiographic, treadmill, and exercise electrocardiographic parameters. J Am Soc Echocardiogr 2003; 16:318–325.

53. Marwick TH, Shaw L, Case C, et al. Clinical and economic impact of exercise electrocardiography and exercise echocardiography in clinical practice. Eur Heart J 2003; 24:1153–1163.

54. Chuah SC, Pellikka PA, Roger VL, et al. Role of dobutamine stress echocardiography in predicting outcome in 860 patients with known or suspected coronary artery disease. Circulation 1998; 97:1474–1480.

55. Marwick TH, Case C, Sawada S, et al. Prediction of mortality using dobutamine echocardiography. J Am Coll Cardiol 2001; 37:754–760.

56. Sicari R, Pasanisi E, Venneri L, et al. Stress echo results predict mortality: A large-scale multicenter prospective international study. J Am Coll Cardiol 2003; 41:589–595.

57. Geleijnse ML, Elhendy A, van Domburg RT, et al. Cardiac imaging for risk stratification with dobutamine-atropine stress testing in patients with chest pain. Echocardiography, perfusion scintigraphy, or both? Circulation 1997; 96:137–147.

58. Shaw U, Peterson ED, Kesler K, et al. A metaanalysis of predischarge risk stratification after acute myocardial infarction with stress electrocardiographic, myocardial perfusion, and ventricular function imaging. Am J Cardiol 1996; 78:1327–1337.

59. Carlos ME, Smart SC, Wynsen JC, et al. Dobutamine stress echocardiography for risk stratification after myocardial infarction. Circulation 1997; 95:1402–1410.

60. Picano E, Sicari R, Landi P, et al. Prognostic value of myocardial viability in medically treated patients with global left ventricular dysfunction early after an acute uncomplicated myocardial infarction: A dobutamine stress echocardiographic study. Circulation 1998; 98:1078–1084.

61. Sicari R, Landi P, Picano E, et al. Exercise-electrocardiography and/or pharmacological stress echocardiography for non-invasive risk stratification early after uncomplicated myocardial infarction: A prospective international large scale multicentre study. Eur Heart J 2002; 23:1030–1037.

62. Poldermans D, Arnese M, Fioretti PM, et al. Improved cardiac risk stratification in major vascular surgery with dobutamine-atropine stress echocardiography. J Am Coll Cardiol 1995; 26:648–653.

63. Shaw LI, Eagle KA, Gersh BI, et al. Meta-analysis of intravenous dipyridamole-thallium-201 imaging (1985 to 1994) and dobutamine echocardiography (1991 to 1994) for risk stratification before vascular surgery. J Am Coll Cardiol 1996; 27:787–798.

64. Pasquet A, D'Hondt AM, Verhelst R, et al. Comparison of dipyridamole stress echocardiography and perfusion scintigraphy for cardiac risk stratification in vascular surgery patients. Am J Cardiol 1998; 82:1468–1474.

65. Firoozan S, Wei K, Linka A, et al. A canine model of chronic ischemic cardiomyopathy: Characterization of regional flow-function relations. Am J Physiol 1999; 276:H446–H455.

66. Lieberman AN, Weiss JL, Jugdutt BI, et al. Relationship of regional wall motion and thickening to the extent of myocardial infarction in the dog. Circulation 1981; 63:739–746.

67. Marzullo P, Parodi O, Reisenhofer B, et al. Value of rest thallium-201/technetium-99 m sestamibi scans and dobutamine echocardiography for detecting myocardial viability. Am J Cardiol 1993; 71:166–172.

68. Charney R, Schwinger ME, Chun J, et al. Dobutamine echocardiography and resting-redistribution thallium-201 scintigraphy predicts recovery of hibernating myocardium after coronary revascularization. Am Heart J 1994; 128:864–869.

69. Qureshi U, Nagueh SF, Afridi I, et al. Dobutamine echocardiography and quantitative rest-redistribution 201T1 tomography in myocardial hibernation. Relation of contractile reserve to uptake and comparative prediction of recovery of function. Circulation 1997; 95:626–635.

70. Nagueh SF, Vaduganathan P, Ali N, et al. Identification of hibernating myocardium: Comparative accuracy of myocardial contrast echocardiography, rest-redistribution thallium-201 tomography and dobutamine echocardiography. J Am Coll Cardiol 1997; 29:985–993.

71. Afridi I, Kleiman NS, Raizner AE, et al. Dobutamine echocardiography in myocardial hibernation: Optimal dose and accuracy in predicting recovery of ventricular function after coronary angioplasty. Circulation 1995; 91:663–670.

72. Bax JJ, Poldermans D, Elhendy A, et al. Sensitivity, specificity, and predictive accuracies of various noninvasive techniques for detecting hibernating myocardium. Curr Probl Cardiol 2001; 26:141–186.

73. Cwajg JM, Cwajg E, Nagueh SF, et al. End-diastolic wall thickness as a predictor of recovery of function in myocardial hibernation: Relation to rest-redistribution T1-201 tomography and dobutamine stress echocardiography. J Am Coll Cardiol 2000; 35:1152–1161.

74. Zaglavara T, Pillay T, Karvounis H, et al. Detection of myocardial viability by dobutamine stress echocardiography: Incremental value of diastolic wall thickness measurement. Heart 2005; 91(5):613–617.

75. Afridi I, Grayburn PA, Panza JA, et al. Myocardial viability during dobutamine echocardiography predicts survival in patients with coronary artery disease and severe left ventricular systolic dysfunction. J Am Coll Cardiol 1998; 32:921–926.

76. Cornel JH, Bax JJ, Elhendy A, et al. Biphasic response to dobutamine predicts improvement of global left ventricular function after surgical revascularization in

patients with stable coronary artery disease: Implications of time course of recovery on diagnostic accuracy. J Am Coll Cardiol 1998; 31:1002–1010.

77. Ragosta M, Beller GA, Watson DD, et al. Quantitative planar rest-redistribution 201T1 imaging in detection of myocardial viability and prediction of improvement in left ventricular function after coronary bypass surgery in patients with severely depressed left ventricular function. Circulation 1993; 87:1630–1641.

78. Pasquet A, Lauer MS, Williams MJ, et al. Prediction of global left ventricular function after bypass surgery in patients with severe left ventricular dysfunction. Impact of pre-operative myocardial function, perfusion, and metabolism. Eur Heart J 2000; 21:125–136.

79. Ailman KG, Shaw LI, Hachamovitch R, et al. Myocardial viability testing and impact of revascularization on prognosis in patients with coronary artery disease and left ventricular dysfunction: A meta-analysis. J Am Coll Cardiol 2002; 39:1151–1158.

80. Meluzin J, Cerny J, Frelich MS, et al. Prognostic value of the amount of dysfunctional but viable myocardium in revascularized patients with coronary artery disease and left ventricular dysfunction. J Am Coil Cardiol 1998; 32:912–920.

81. Marwick TH, Shaw U, Lauer MS, et al. The noninvasive prediction of cardiac mortality in men and women with known or suspected coronary artery disease. Economics of Non-invasive Diagnosis (END) Study Group. Am J Med 1999; 106:172–178.

82. Marwick TH, Mehta R, Arheart K, et al. Use of exercise echocardiography for prognostic evaluation of patients with known or suspected coronary artery disease. J Am Coll Cardiol 1997; 30:83–90.

83. Picano E, Seven S, Michelassi C, et al. Prognostic importance of dipyridamole echocardiography test in coronary artery disease. Circulation 1989; 80:450–457.

84. Marwick TH, Case C, Sawada S, et al. Use of stress echocardiography to predict mortality in patients with diabetes and known or suspected coronary artery disease. Diabetes Care 2002; 25:1042–1048.

85. Pryor DB, Shaw L, McCants CB, et al. Value of the history and physical in identifying patients at increased risk for coronary artery disease. Ann Intern Med 1993; 118:81–90.

86. Berman DS, Hachamovitch R, Kiat H, et al. Incremental value of prognostic testing in patients with known or suspected ischemic heart disease: A basis for optimal utilization of exercise technetium-99 m sestamibi myocardial perfusion single-photon emission computed tomography. J Am Coll Cardiol 1995; 26:639–647.

87. Patterson RE, Eisner RL, Horowitz SF. Comparison of cost-effectiveness and utility of exercise ECG, single photon emission computed tomography, positron emission tomography, and coronary angiography for diagnosis of coronary artery disease. Circulation 1995; 91:54–65.

88. Kuntz KM, Fleischmann KE, Hunink MG, et al. Cost-effectiveness of diagnostic strategies for patients with chest pain. Ann Intern Med 1999; 130:709–718.

89. Shaw LJ, Hachamovitch R, Berman DS, et al. The economic consequences of available diagnostic and prognostic strategies for the evaluation of stable angina patients: An observational assessment of the value of precatheterization ischemia. Economics of Noninvasive Diagnosis (END) Multicenter Study Group. J Am Coll Cardiol 1999; 33:661–669.

90. Underwood SR, Godman B, Salyani S, et al. Economics of myocardial perfusion imaging in Europe—The EMPIRE study. Eur Heart J 1999; 20:157–166.

91. Shaw L, Marwick T, Berman D, et al. Incremental cost-effectiveness of exercise echocardiography vs. SPECT imaging for the evaluation of stable chest pain. Eur Heart J 2006; 27:2448–2458.

92. King SB III, Smith SC Jr, Hirshfeld JW Jr, et al. 2007 Focused Update of the ACC/AHA/SCAI 2005 Guideline Update for Percutaneous Coronary Intervention: A report of the American College of Cardiology/American Heart Association Task Force on Practice Guidelines. Circulation 2008; 117(2):261–295 [Epub Dec. 13, 2007].

13 Training in Stress Echocardiography

Frank A. Flachskampf

Medizinische Klinik 2, University of Erlangen, Erlangen, Germany

Stress echocardiography "combines the most difficult part of echocardiography, the assessment of wall motion abnormalities, with the most boring part of cardiology, the performance of stress tests" (A. E. Weyman). Training therefore is of paramount importance in this particular field, perhaps even more so than in other subspecialties of echocardiography. Stress echocardiography is an advanced technique and requires experience in transthoracic echocardiography, because the recognition of range and limits of normalcy is critical in interpreting stress echo images. The trainee should learn to properly acquire the images, to handle the software for storage and display of recorded images, and to systematically interpret the stress test comparing baseline and stress images segment by segment. Typical errors such as acquisition of nonstandard cross sections due to time pressure, false triggering due to ECG artifacts, or arrhythmias leading to uninterpretable cine-loops, etc., should be recognized and corrected. Importantly, the trainee must learn to recognize large inducible wall motion abnormalities that should lead to termination of the study.

The following minimum training requirements have been proposed:

* EAE (1): proficiency (preferably accreditation) in transthoracic echocardiography, 100 supervised studies for trainees in stress echo, 100 studies per year for maintenance of competence.
* American College of Cardiology and American Society of Echocardiography 2003 (2): level 2 training in transthoracic echocardiography (minimum of 6 months of echo training and 300 studies interpreted) and 100 stress echos read under supervision to achieve competence and reading 100 stress echos per year, as well as continuing medical education credits to maintain competence (and performing 10 per month for a sonographer to maintain competence).

Besides, the ability to manage the inevitably occurring, if rare, complications of stress tests is crucial. A physician trained in resuscitation and intensive care has to be physically present in the laboratory when a stress test is done. Besides the necessary hardware, which is covered elsewhere in this book, a "standard operating procedure" for the case of an emergency needs to be in place and thoroughly rehearsed by all involved. This includes how to obtain immediate (within seconds) help from other medical personnel.

Ideally, a laboratory performing stress echos should regularly review studies and compare them to coronary angiography findings. Such sessions should be attended by all persons involved in stress echo to provide feedback and discuss practices, and thus to assure quality. Feedback is necessary even for experienced echocardiographers, and exposure to stress echo seems to be necessary to

177

maintain expertise. As much information from angiography should be obtained as possible; ideally, the angiograms should be reviewed, too, because written report often do not provide sufficient detail, for example, about the size of a vessel, stenosed branches, collaterals, etc.

The "importance of being expert" has been demonstrated by Picano et al. (3). Although newer technology (harmonic imaging, higher frame rates, improved transducers, digital storage and display) certainly has improved image quality and facilitated stress echocardiography, the task is still a difficult one, and the patient population has, at least in many places, become older and sicker, with more patients with previous infarction, in heart failure, and with concomitant diseases. In spite of several techniques which enable a degree of quantification in wall motion assessment, in general the visual assessment is still decisive for calling a study normal or abnormal. In fact, a study (4) showed that many so-called false-negative studies even after careful quantitation remain negative, because no ischemia was elicited by the applied stress. This possibility should always be kept in mind when comparing stress test results to an angiographic standard.

REFERENCES

1. Sicari R, Nihoyannopoulos P, Evangelista A, et al. Stress echocardiography expert consensus statement: European Association of Echocardiography (EAE) (a registered branch of the ESC). Eur J Echocardiogr 2008; 9:415–437.
2. Quinones MA, Douglas PS, Foster E, et al. ACC/AHA clinical competence statement on echocardiography: A report of the American College of Cardiology/American Heart Association/American College of Physicians—American Society of Internal Medicine Task Force on Clinical Competence (Committee on Echocardiography). J Am Coll Cardiol 2003; 41:687–708.
3. Picano E, Lattanzi F, Orlandini A, et al. Stress echocardiography and the human factor: The importance of being expert. J Am Coll Cardiol 1991; 17:666–669.
4. Yuda S, Fang ZY, Leano R, et al. Is quantitative interpretation likely to increase sensitivity of dobutamine stress echocardiography? A study of false-negative results. J Am Soc Echocardiogr 2004; 17:448–453.

Landmark Articles with Short Comments

Frank A. Flachskampf

Medizinische Klinik 2, University of Erlangen, Erlangen, Germany

The following is a list of important publications in the field of stress echocardiography. Such a list is necessarily subjective and this compilation by no means claims to be exhaustive, regardless of which criteria for "importance" are applied. A search in Medline's PubMed facility revealed 6912 papers on "stress echocardiography" in September 2009. Nevertheless, the author believes that the cited papers are indeed instructive and represent important progress in the field. They are arranged thematically despite some topic overlap.

I. EXERCISE ECHOCARDIOGRAPHY

Wann LS, Faris JV, Childress RH, et al. Exercise cross-sectional echocardiography in ischemic heart disease. Circulation 1979; 60:1300–1308.

Commentary: This is the first major report on stress echo using 2D echo (previous reports used M-mode echocardiography). Twenty-eight patients were studied before and during bicycle exercise by 2D echo. Interpretable images were acquired in 20/28 (71%) patients, with good sensitivity for coronary artery disease. The authors concluded, in a still valid statement, that stress echo was "technically difficult but feasible."

Quinones MA, Verani MS, Haichin RM, et al. Exercise echocardiography versus 201Tl single-photon emission computed tomography in evaluation of coronary artery disease. Analysis of 292 patients. Circulation 1992; 85:1026–1031.

Commentary: This is a large correlative study of exercise stress echo and Thallium-SPECT nuclear perfusion imaging in 292 patients. Diagnostic accuracy in this study was very similar for both methods and depended on the number of diseased vessels.

Arnese M, Salustri A, Fioretti PM, et al. Quantitative angiographic measurements of isolated left anterior descending coronary artery stenosis. Correlation with exercise echocardiography and technetium-99 m 2-methoxy isobutyl isonitrile single-photon emission computed tomography. J Am Coll Cardiol 1995; 25:1486–1491.

Commentary: The universal cutoff for coronary artery diameter stenosis to become significant is usually set at 50%, although some authors use 70%. In this study, reversing the usual viewpoint, the authors looked at patients with angiographically known left anterior descending stenosis to evaluate which degree of stenosis best predicted a positive dobutamine stress echo or MIBI-SPECT. The result was a diameter stenosis of 52% for echo and 49% for nuclear imaging.

Marwick TH, Mehta R, Arheart K, et al. Use of exercise echocardiography for prognostic evaluation of patients with known or suspected coronary artery disease. J Am Coll Cardiol 1997; 30:83–90.

Commentary: A total of 500 patients underwent exercise stress echo; those having revascularization over the next 3 months ($n = 16$) were excluded. Stress echo results and ability to exercise were independent prognostic predictors, showing the incremental value over stress echo to classic exercise ECG.

Arruda AM, Das MK, Roger VL, et al. Prognostic value of exercise echocardiography in 2632 patients > or = 65 years of age. J Am Coll Cardiol 2001; 37:1036–1041.

Commentary: This study documents the prognostic value of exercise echocardiography in the elderly. A total of 2632 patients 65 years or older were followed over an average of 3 years. Exercise stress echo results provided additional independent prognostic value in this important subgroup. Interestingly, this was a relatively low-risk group of elderly patients, probably because they were selected to be able to exercise.

Elhendy A, Arruda AM, Mahoney DW, et al. Prognostic stratification of diabetic patients by exercise echocardiography. J Am Coll Cardiol 2001; 37:1551–1557.

Commentary: This study documents the prognostic value of exercise echocardiography in diabetic patients, which is similar to that in nondiabetic patients. A normal exercise echo predicted a very low cardiac death/myocardial infarction rate (0% in the first and 7.6% after five years).

Marwick TH, Case C, Vasey C, et al. Prediction of mortality by exercise echocardiography. A strategy for combination with the Duke treadmill score. Circulation 2001; 103:2566–2571.

Commentary: In a collective of 5375 patients undergoing exercise echocardiography, follow-up was obtained over a mean of 5.5 years. A normal stress echo identified patients with a low mortality of 1% per year. Importantly, this study shows in a very substantial number of patients that exercise echo is not inferior to perfusion scintigraphy in risk stratifying patients; it had long been a claim of nuclear medicine to have a better-documented prognostic power than stress echo.

Metz LD, Beattie M, Hom R, et al. The prognostic value of normal exercise myocardial perfusion imaging and exercise echocardiography: A meta-analysis. J Am Coll Cardiol 2007; 49:227–237.

Commentary: Similar to the article by Marwick et al. (2001), this meta-analysis pooling over 8000 patients shows the excellent negative predictive value of a normal exercise stress echo. A negative exercise stress echo predicted an annual mortality of 1% or combined rate of myocardial infarction or cardiac death of ≤1%, hence conferring a low cardiovascular risk status to such patients. These results indicate a very similar prognostic power for exercise echocardiography as for nuclear perfusion stress tests. Clearly, however, these results have to be understood in the context of patient selection—neither the very low-risk (e.g., the asymptomatic young) nor the very high-risk patients (e.g., those with severe symptoms) usually are stress tested, nor should they be. Therefore, these data apply to patients at intermediate pretest cardiovascular risk.

Bouzas-Mosquera A, Peteiro J, Alvarez-García N, Broullón FJ, Mosquera VX, García-Bueno L, Ferro L, Castro-Beiras A. Prediction of mortality and major cardiac events by exercise echocardiography in patients with normal exercise electrocardiographic testing. J Am Coll Cardiol 2009;53:1981–1990.

Commentary: This paper is rather unique since it focusses on patients who had a normal treadmill ECG test (no angina, no ST depression) and simultaneously, stress echocardiography during the treadmill test. The authors followed 4004 such patients evaluated for chest pain and found that one in six of them had an ischemic stress echo response, which predicted a doubling of the rate of death or myocardial infarction over the next five years; for patients with a low Duke treadmill score, this rate was even fivefold higher. The paper shows convincingly that routine exercise ECG is suboptimal for prognosis and that exercise stress echo is well feasible on the treadmill (at least in experienced hands) and has much higher diagnostic power.

II. DOBUTAMINE STRESS ECHOCARDIOGRAPHY

Berthe C, Pierard LA, Hiernaux M, et al. Predicting the extent and location of coronary artery disease in acute myocardial infarction by echocardiography during dobutamine infusion. Am J Cardiol 1986; 58:1167–1172.

Commentary: This is the first major report on the use of dobutamine for stress echocardiography. Thirty patients underwent the test after acute myocardial infarction, and a sensitivity of 85% was seen for the detection of "multivessel disease."

Sawada SG, Segar DS, Ryan T, et al. Echocardiographic detection of coronary artery disease during dobutamine infusion. Circulation 1991; 83:1605–1614.

Commentary: In this early experience with dobutamine stress echo, digital capture of cine-loops was used for evaluation of wall motion, a technique not generally utilized before. The careful evaluation of 103 patients undergoing coronary angiography yielded a high sensitivity (89%) for coronary artery disease. The prevalence of disease was high in this population (81 out of 105), and half of the patients had resting wall motion abnormalities.

Marwick T, Willemart B, D'Hondt AM, et al. Selection of the optimal nonexercise stress for the evaluation of ischemic regional myocardial dysfunction and malperfusion. Comparison of dobutamine and adenosine using echocardiography and 99mTc-MIBI single photon emission computed tomography. Circulation 1993; 87:345–354.

Commentary: This study compared the diagnostic accuracy of two pharmacologic stressors, dobutamine and adenosine, and two imaging modalities, stress echo and MIBI-SPECT nuclear imaging, in the same 97 patients (compared to coronary angiography). The data show an unacceptably low sensitivity of adenosine stress echo, and similar accuracies (sensitivities 80–86% and specificities 71–82%) for dobutamine echo or nuclear imaging, as well as for adenosine nuclear imaging.

Bach DS, Muller DW, Gros BJ, et al. False positive dobutamine stress echocardiograms: Characterization of clinical, echocardiographic and angiographic findings. J Am Coll Cardiol 1994; 24:928–933.

Commentary: An interesting early study of false positivity in dobutamine stress echo. Basal segments were most often falsely assumed to be ischemic, a finding reproduced later by many other investigators. The authors also point out that some angiographically intermediate stenoses may actually be underestimated by angiography rather than "overestimated" by stress echo.

Poldermans D, Fioretti PM, Boersma E, et al. Dobutamine-atropine stress echocardiography and clinical data for predicting late cardiac events in patients with suspected coronary artery disease. Am J Med 1994; 97:119–125.

Commentary: A total of 430 stable chest pain patients were evaluated by dobutamine stress echo and results were related to prognosis over a mean follow-up of 17 months. New inducible wall motion abnormalities were predictive of death or a combination endpoint of death, infarction, and revascularization, independently of other clinical variables.

Picano E, Mathias W Jr, Pingitore A, et al. Safety and tolerability of dobutamine-atropine stress echocardiography: A prospective, multicentre study. Echo Dobutamine International Cooperative Study Group. Lancet 1994; 344:1190–1192.

Commentary: In almost 3000 dobutamine stress echos from several centers, 14 (5 per 1000) life-threatening side effects were seen: ventricular tachycardia or fibrillation, myocardial infarction, and severe hypotension.

Bartunek J, Marwick TH, Rodrigues AC, et al. Dobutamine-induced wall motion abnormalities: Correlations with myocardial fractional flow reserve and quantitative coronary angiography. J Am Coll Cardiol 1996; 27:1429–1436.

Commentary: This important study compared findings on dobutamine stress echo to quantitative angiography and fractional flow reserve measured by the pressure wire. Seventy-five patients with normal left ventricular function and coronary artery disease participated. As one would expect, although there was a correlation between inducible dyssynergy and degree of stenosis, this correlation was modest ($r = 0.68$), and marked scattering was observed. Nevertheless, sensitivity and specificity of stress echo for >50% stenosis were 83% and 80%, respectively. Sensitivity and specificity of stress echo to predict a myocardial fractional flow reserve <75% were 76% and 97%. Stress echo was less accurate to detect stenoses in smaller vessels with a reference diameter <2.6 mm.

Secknus MA, Marwick TH. Evolution of dobutamine echocardiography protocols and indications: Safety and side effects in 3011 studies over 5 years. J Am
Coll Cardiol 1997; 29:1234–1240.

Commentary: In this single-center study similar to Picano's 1994 multicenter report, 9 (0.3%) "serious complications" occurred (ventricular tachycardia,
hypotension, severe prolonged myocardial ischemia).

Geleijnse ML, Elhendy A, van Domburg RT, et al. Cardiac imaging for risk stratification with dobutamine-atropine stress testing in patients with chest pain.
Echocardiography, perfusion scintigraphy, or both? Circulation 1997; 96:137–
147.

Commentary: This study analyzed the predictive value of dobutamine stress
echo and MIBI-SPECT performed in parallel in 220 patients with chest pain. Both
techniques were found to have similar prognostic value, with ischemia and/or
scar predicting higher mortality and myocardial infarction.

Poldermans D, Fioretti PM, Boersma E, et al. Long-term prognostic value of
dobutamine-atropine stress echocardiography in 1737 patients with known
or suspected coronary artery disease: A single-center experience. Circulation
1999; 99:757–762.

Commentary: Follow-up was obtained in 1659 patients after exclusion of 74
patients revascularized within 3 months after the test. Dobutamine stress echo
findings (both presence and extent of ischemia) risk-stratified patients well. Similar to other large studies, the annual cardiac death or infarction rate after a negative stress echo was low, 1.3%.

Marwick TH, Case C, Sawada S, et al. Prediction of mortality using dobutamine
echocardiography. J Am Coll Cardiol 2001; 37:754–760.

Commentary: A total of 3156 stable patients were evaluated for coronary artery
disease. During a mean follow-up of 4 years, the results of dobutamine stress
echocardiography strongly predicted prognosis, with the worst prognosis in
patients exhibiting both scars and ischemia, followed by scar or ischemia, and a
good prognosis (1% cardiac mortality per year) for patients with a normal dobutamine stress echo.

III. DIPYRIDAMOLE STRESS ECHOCARDIOGRAPHY

Picano E, Severi S, Michelassi C, et al. Prognostic importance of dipyridamole-
echocardiography test in coronary artery disease. Circulation 1989; 80:450–457.

Commentary: This was the first study to show in a large cohort of patients
($n = 539$) that a positive dipyridamole echo is a marker of adverse prognosis
regarding the hard endpoints death and myocardial infarction. Follow-up time
was 3 years.

Picano E, Marini C, Pirelli S, et al. Safety of intravenous high-dose dipyridamole echocardiography. The Echo-Persantine International Cooperative
Study Group. Am J Cardiol 1992; 70:252–258.

Commentary: In 10,451 dipyridamole stress echos, 7 "major adverse reactions" were seen (0.1%). One of these, with prolonged asystole and subsequent myocardial infarction led to death. Other major adverse reactions were myocardial infarction, ventricular tachycardia, and pulmonary edema. In most minor adverse reactions, dipyridamole effects were promptly reversed by aminophylline.

Picano E, Landi P, Bolognese L, et al. Prognostic value of dipyridamole echocardiography early after uncomplicated myocardial infarction: A large-scale, multicenter trial. The EPIC Study Group. Am J Med 1993; 95:608–618.

Commentary: In this multicenter study from 11 institutions, 925 patients after acute myocardial infarction were evaluated by dipyridamole stress echo and followed-up for 14 months. Presence, severity, and extent of new wall motion abnormalities under dipyridamole were predictive of death, new angina, or reinfarction.

Cortigiani L, Rigo F, Gherardi S, Sicari R, Galderisi M, Bovenzi F, Picano E. Additional prognostic value of coronary flow reserve in diabetic and nondiabetic patients with negative dipyridamole stress echocardiography by wall motion criteria. J Am Coll Cardiol 2007; 50:1354–1361.

Commentary: 1130 patients who did not show new wall motion abnormalities on dipyridamole stress echo had simultaneous coronary flow velocity reserve assessment by transthoracic Doppler examination of the left anterior descending. An impaired coronary flow velocity reserve (≤ 2) occurred in 27% of these patients and independently of other characteristics predicted adverse events.

IV. STRESS ECHO FOR PREOPERATIVE CARDIOVASCULAR RISK ASSESSMENT

Shaw LJ, Eagle KA, Gersh BJ, et al. Meta-analysis of intravenous dipyridamole-thallium-201 imaging (1985 to 1994) and dobutamine echocardiography (1991 to 1994) for risk stratification before vascular surgery. J Am Coll Cardiol 1996; 27:787–798.

Commentary: This meta-analysis of dobutamine stress echo and dipyridamole nuclear perfusion scanning for risk stratification in patients before vascular surgery showed a very high negative predictive value of a normal dobutamine stress echo in a pooled analysis of 445 patients for perioperative ischemic cardiac events (99%). Understandably, the positive predictive value for such events was quite low, but it is the negative value (the probability that the patient will fare well perioperatively if he has a normal stress test) that matters here, because positive stress tests will have individualized clinical consequences difficult to analyze in a summary way.

Sicari R, Ripoli A, Picano E, et al. Perioperative prognostic value of dipyridamole echocardiography in vascular surgery: A large-scale multicenter study in 509 patients. EPIC (Echo Persantine International Cooperative) Study Group. Circulation 1999; 100(19 Suppl.):II269–II274.

Commentary: Dipyridamole stress echo was successfully used in this multicenter study. The negative predictive value of stress echo was 99%, well comparable to that of dobutamine stress echo.

Poldermans D, Boersma E, Bax JJ, et al. The effect of bisoprolol on perioperative mortality and myocardial infarction in high-risk patients undergoing vascular surgery. Dutch Echocardiographic Cardiac Risk Evaluation Applying Stress Echocardiography Study Group. N Engl J Med 1999; 341:1789–1794.

Boersma E, Poldermans D, Bax JJ, et al.; DECREASE Study Group (Dutch Echocardiographic Cardiac Risk Evaluation Applying Stress Echocardiography). Predictors of cardiac events after major vascular surgery: Role of clinical characteristics, dobutamine echocardiography, and beta-blocker therapy. JAMA 2001; 285:1865–1873.

Commentary: In an interesting twist, the Dutch group of Poldermans et al. showed that use of β-blockers (bisoprolol or metoprolol to achieve a resting heart rate of about 60/min) massively reduced the perioperative complication rate (death and myocardial infarction) in patients with a positive (pathologic) dobutamine echo result before vascular surgery (3.4% in the β-blocker group vs. 34% in the non–β-blocker group). The authors then showed in the next study that stress echo testing in patients on β-blockers who undergo vascular surgery does not add substantial information, if patients are in an intermediate-risk group; however, dobutamine stress echo in high-risk patients appeared still to be useful to identify those patients who had large inducible ischemia (more than four segments with new wall motion abnormalities) and therefore seemed to profit from preoperative revascularization.

V. ASSESSMENT OF VIABILITY

Pierard LA, De Landsheere CM, Berthe C, et al. Identification of viable myocardium by echocardiography during dobutamine infusion in patients with myocardial infarction after thrombolytic therapy: Comparison with positron emission tomography. J Am Coll Cardiol 1990; 15:1021–1031.

Commentary: In this pioneering study, 17 patients after anterior myocardial infarction and thrombolysis were studied by dobutamine stress echo and positron emission tomography and compared to a follow-up evaluation 9 months later, showing a good diagnostic accuracy of regional contractile reserve under dobutamine stimulation for functional recovery. This was the first clinical study showing the use of dobutamine stress echo for detecting viability (here still called "stunning" regardless of the time course) after myocardial infarction.

Afridi I, Kleiman NS, Raizner AE, et al. Dobutamine echocardiography in myocardial hibernation: Optimal dose and accuracy in predicting recovery of ventricular function after coronary angioplasty. Circulation 1995; 91:663–670.

Commentary: This is a very careful study of the response of dysfunctional myocardium to dobutamine stimulation, validating the use of dobutamine stress echo for the detection of viable, hibernating myocardium. Twenty patients were studied before and after angioplasty in small dobutamine dosage increments. The dose at which improvement was most prevalent in the presence of viable myocardium was 7.5 μg/kg/min. If a biphasic response was present, the ischemic phase occurred at dosages of 20 μg/kg/min or higher.

Arnese M, Cornel JH, Salustri A, et al. Prediction of improvement of regional left ventricular function after surgical revascularization. A comparison of low-dose dobutamine echocardiography with 201Tl single-photon emission computed tomography. Circulation 1995; 91:2748–2752.

Commentary: This study compared low-dose dobutamine stress echo (10 μg/min/kg) with thallium reinjection imaging to detect viable myocardium in patients with left ventricular systolic impairment undergoing bypass surgery. Results were compared to postoperative functional improvement. The data show a much better diagnostic accuracy for dobutamine echo, because thallium imaging tended to overestimate residual viability (low positive predictive value, high negative predictive value). The data have to be interpreted in the context of the definition of "viability"; this study focussed on segments that improved in contractile function after revascularization. There may be some viability in segments which do not improve after revascularization, and patients may profit from such viability (e.g., perhaps in the occurrence of sudden death or with regard to left ventricular remodeling) even if regional and global left ventricular function does not improve.

Hoffer EP, Dewe W, Celentano C, et al. Low-level exercise echocardiography detects contractile reserve and predicts reversible dysfunction after acute myocardial infarction: Comparison with low-dose dobutamine echocardiography. J Am Coll Cardiol 1999; 34:989–997.

Commentary: This is the first study showing that low-level exercise can be used to elicit a contractile response, similar to low-dose dobutamine, in dyssynergic, but viable myocardium.

Underwood SR, Bax JJ, vom Dahl J, et al; Study Group of the European Society of Cardiology Imaging techniques for the assessment of myocardial hibernation. Report of a Study Group of the European Society of Cardiology. Eur Heart J 2004; 25:815–836 [Erratum in: Eur Heart J 2004; 25:2176].

Commentary: A review of the available literature by a study group of the European Society of Cardiology, which systematically evaluated the literature on different modalities to diagnose hibernating myocardium. This study came to a similar conclusion as the paper of Arnese et al., with low-dose dobutamine stress echo and nuclear imaging as the two primary techniques with similar diagnostic accuracy, echo having a slightly higher positive predictive accuracy and slightly lower negative predictive value than nuclear scanning.

VI. MISCELLANEOUS ISSUES

Picano E, Lattanzi F, Orlandini A, et al. Stress echocardiography and the human factor: The importance of being expert. J Am Coll Cardiol 1991; 17:666–669.

Commentary: This observation documents the learning curve in echocardiography. The authors found that after reading 100 stress echos, stress echo beginners (although with good knowledge in conventional echocardiography) approached the diagnostic accuracy of experts, while accuracy was substantially lower at the outset.

Beleslin BD, Ostojic M, Stepanovic J, et al. Stress echocardiography in the detection of myocardial ischemia. Head-to-head comparison of exercise, dobutamine, and dipyridamole tests. Circulation 1994; 90:1168–1176.

Commentary: In this study, the same 136 patients underwent exercise, dobutamine, and dipyridamole stress echo; results were compared to coronary angiography. There was a very high incidence of significant coronary artery disease in this patient group (87%). Sensitivity was highest for exercise, followed by dobutamine and dipyridamole (88%, 82%, 76%, respectively), while specificities were 82%, 77%, and 94%, respectively. The study is unique in that it compares all three major types of stress echo in the same patients.

Mairesse GH, Marwick T, Arnese M, et al. Improved identification of coronary artery disease in patients with left bundle branch block by use of dobutamine stress echocardiography and comparison with myocardial perfusion tomography. Am J Cardiol 1995; 76:321–325.

Commentary: This study compared the diagnostic accuracy of dobutamine stress echo and with MIBI-SPECT in 24 patients with left bundle branch block, a well-known problem in the interpretation of stress tests. Twelve of the patients had critical left anterior descending stenosis, while the rest did not. Stress echo, by focussing on wall thickening, achieved a sensitivity of 83% and a specificity of 92%, while scintigraphy was always pathologic for yielding a sensitivity of 100%, but a specificity of 0%.

Hoffmann R, Lethen H, Marwick T, et al. Analysis of interinstitutional observer agreement in the interpretation of dobutamine stress echocardiography. J Am Coll Cardiol 1996; 27:330–336.

Hoffmann R, Marwick TH, Poldermans D, et al. Refinements in stress echocardiographic techniques improve inter-institutional agreement in interpretation of dobutamine stress echocardiograms. Eur Heart J 2002; 23:821–829.

Commentary: In the first study, interobserver variability was assessed by comparing the evaluation of 150 dobutamine stress echos by five different centers. Intercenter concordance was relatively low (kappa 0.37, majority agreement 73%). The follow up study involved six centers and again a set of 150 dobutamine stress echos read independently at each center. This time, digital capture, and storage as well as harmonic imaging were used and a set of rules was jointly followed such as disregarding hypokinesia occurring exclusively in the basal inferior or basal septum. A clear improvement of the kappa value to 0.55 resulted, showing progress in the diagnostic accuracy of stress echo over the intervening 6 years.

VII. NEW TECHNIQUES: TISSUE DOPPLER, DEFORMATION IMAGING, CONTRAST ECHO, 3D

Voigt JU, Exner B, Schmiedehausen K, et al. Strain rate imaging during dobutamine stress echocardiography provides objective evidence of inducible
ischemia. Circulation 2003; 107:2120–2126.

Commentary: Strain and strain rate was measured during dobutamine stress
echo in 44 patients and compared to wall motion assessment, concomitant
nuclear imaging, and coronary angiography. Strain and strain rate were reduced
and the ratio of postsystolic shortening to maximal strain was increased in
ischemic segments, thus moderately improving stress echo sensitivity. The study
shows that there is an incremental diagnostic value—particularly in segments
where visual assessment is ambiguous—to using deformation imaging to detect
inducible ischemia.

Madler CF, Payne N, Wilkenshoff U, et al; Myocardial Doppler in Stress Echocardiography (MYDISE) Study Investigators. Non-invasive diagnosis of coronary
artery disease by quantitative stress echocardiography: Optimal diagnostic
models using off-line tissue Doppler in the MYDISE study. Eur Heart J 2003;
24:1584–1594.

Commentary: This was the first larger study to examine the value of tissue
velocity data for the diagnosis of ischemia by stress echo. It is an eight-center
study of dobutamine stress echo in 289 patients without previous myocardial
infarction. Except for the normal control group all had coronary angiography.
Peak systolic tissue velocities were found predictive of ≥50% major coronary
artery diameter stenosis, with sensitivities and specificities (calculated per coronary artery) between 60% and 69%. Better results, however, were obtained
using a multivariate regression analysis of the data in which a different equa-
tion was constructed for each coronary artery for the prediction of critical
stenosis, taking into account also age, gender, and peak heart rate. Sensitivities and specificities (calculated by diseased artery) of these models lie between
80% and 93%. No comparison with qualitative stress echo reading was undertaken. The study shows that stress echo response can be objectively documented
by tissue velocities, but interpretation of these data is complex, since there is
no simple and reliable cutoff of myocardial velocities to diagnose inducible
wall motion abnormalities. In particular, it was not clear how much of an
improvement in practical terms this constitutes over classic stress echo interpretation.

Hanekom L, Jenkins C, Jeffries L, et al. Incremental value of strain rate analysis
as an adjunct to wall-motion scoring for assessment of myocardial viability
by dobutamine echocardiography: A follow-up study after revascularization.
Circulation 2005; 112:3892–3900.

Commentary: This study for the first time showed in a reasonable number of
patients ($n = 55$) with impaired left ventricular systolic function that deformation parameters add to the detection of viability by dobutamine stress echo. Peak
systolic strain rate and end-systolic strain at low-dose dobutamine improved

detection of viable myocardium by increasing sensitivity compared to visual assessment of wall motion (82% vs. 73%), but did not significantly change specificity (80% vs. 77%). Viability was defined by wall motion improvement 9 months after revascularization.

Elhendy A, O'Leary EL, Xie F, et al. Comparative accuracy of real-time myocardial contrast perfusion imaging and wall motion analysis during dobutamine stress echocardiography for the diagnosis of coronary artery disease. J Am Coll Cardiol 2004; 44:2185–2191.

Tsutsui JM, Elhendy A, Anderson JR, et al. Prognostic value of dobutamine stress myocardial contrast perfusion echocardiography. Circulation 2005; 112:1444–1450.

Commentary: These two landmark papers for the first time reported the results of dobutamine stress myocardial contrast echocardiography for the diagnosis of coronary artery disease. While the first study analyzed 170 patients comparing stress echo to coronary angiography, the second study from the same group looked at the prognostic implications of dobutamine stress contrast echocardiography in 788 patients. Optison® or Definity® were used as left heart contrast agents. Compared to wall motion assessment, assessment of perfusion had a higher sensitivity, with abnormalities occurring before wall motion abnormalities during the stress test, but a lower specificity for the presence of coronary artery disease. On the other hand, impaired coronary perfusion had additive prognostic value.

Matsumura Y, Hozumi T, Arai K, et al. Non-invasive assessment of myocardial ischaemia using new real-time three-dimensional dobutamine stress echocardiography: Comparison with conventional two-dimensional methods. Eur Heart J 2005; 26:1625–1632.

Commentary: This is one of the first studies using real-time 3D stress echocardiography. 3D and 2D dobutamine stress echo results were compared against a "gold standard" of exercise Thallium perfusion imaging. Sensitivity, specificity, and accuracy for the detection of critical coronary stenoses were identical with both echo methods (all $\geq 80\%$); however, acquisition time was shorter by 3D than by 2D echo.

Ishii K, Imai M, Suyama T, Maenaka M, Nagai T, Kawanami M, Seino Y. Exercise-induced post-ischemic left ventricular delayed relaxation or diastolic stunning: is it a reliable marker in detecting coronary artery disease? J Am Coll Cardiol 2009; 53:698–705.

Commentary: This study elegantly used speckle-tracking based deformation imaging ("2D strain") to detect ischemia by identifying delayed relaxation in segments supplied by stenosed coronary arteries up to 10 min after cessation of exercise. This study clearly shows the potential of deformation imaging to detect features of myocardial contraction and relaxation which cannot be seen with the naked eye.

During the last few years, both from the European and the American echo societies recommendations and overviews have been published on stress echo, which are recommended to the reader:

1. Pellikka PA, Nagueh SF, Elhendy AA, Kuehl CA, Sawada SG; American Society of Echocardiography. American Society of Echocardiography recommendations for performance, interpretation, and application of stress echocardiography. J Am Soc Echocardiogr 2007; 20:1021–1041.
2. Sicari R, Nihoyannopoulos P, Evangelista A, et al. Stress echocardiography expert consensus statement: European Association of Echocardiography (EAE) (a registered branch of the ESC). Eur J Echocardiogr 2008; 9:415–437.

Subject Index

16/17-segment model of left ventricle, 26, 54
3D stress echocardiography, 188–90

accreditation, 23–4; *see also* training
accuracy of stress echocardiography and
  different stressors, 60–68, 68–70
adenosine, 7, 13, 14, 14t, 15, 15f, 17f, 45; *see
  also* pharmacological stress echo
akinesia, 2, 6, 31f, 54
American College of Cardiology/American
  Heart Association (ACC/AHA), 121, 143,
  148, 154, 155
American Society of Echocardiography
  (ASE), 22, 101, 121, 128
aminophylline, 13, 43, 44
aortic regurgitation, 124
aortic stenosis, 17, 118, 121–4, 144t, 147
atropine, 27, 62, 63, 67t, 68, 69t, 75t

beta blockers, 40, 42, 48, 57
biphasic response, *see* viability

cardiac risk, 5, 6, 7; *see also* prognosis and risk
  stratification
complications, *see* adverse events
computed tomography, cardiac, 3, 4
contractile reserve in dilated cardiomyopathy,
  131, 133, 134, 135, 136, 138, 139f, 140f
contraindications, 7
contrast echo, agents, protocols, 20, 21, 84–6,
  107–10
Coronary Artery Revascularization
  Prophylaxis (CARP) trial, 154
coronary flow reserve, 3f, 6, 8, 12, 13, 15, 16,
  17f

DECREASE (Dutch Echocardiographic
  Cardiac Risk Evaluation Applying Stress
  Echocardiography), 154, 155t
Definity®, 189

deformation imaging, *see* strain imaging
dilated cardiomyopathy, 131–40
dipyridamole, 1, 7, 13, 14, 15, 17, 43–4; *see also*
  pharmacological stress echo
dobutamine, 1, 7, 12, 13, 14, 15, 16, 17, 40–43;
  viability, 94, 95, 96, 97–103; *see also*
  pharmacological stress echo
dyskinesia, 2, 6, 31f

electrocardiography, stress, 4, 73–4, 147
equipment requirements, 20–22
ergometrine, 12, 13f
ergonovine stress echocardiography, 48
European Association of Echocardiography
  (EAE), 23, 24
European Society of Cardiology (ESC), 8, 121,
  122, 124, 127, 148
exercise (bicycle, treadmill) stress
  echocardiography, 13, 14, 15, 21, 39, 62

false-negative tests, 56, 57, 73, 79
false-positive tests, 56, 57, 73, 79

Goldman risk index, 147, 148

Handgrip, 27
harmonic imaging, 20, 21, 28, 38
hibernation (myocardial), 93, 94, 95; *see also*
  viability
hyperkinesia, 2
hypertrophy (left ventricular), 79
hyperventilation, 13, 49–50
hypokinesia, 2, 31, 54

image acquisition and processing, 27, 37
image interpretation, 29–33, 53–60
ischemia, myocardial, 1, 12, 13f, 14f, 15, 16,
  53–86; *see also* myocardial infarction

left bundle branch block, 57, 79–80, 165t

Printed and bound by CPI Group (UK) Ltd, Croydon, CR0 4YY

23/10/2024

01778266-0001